# Imaging in Trauma

# Imaging in Trauma

**ROBERT COCKS**
*Professor and Director, Accident and Emergency Medicine Academic Unit, Prince of Wales Hospital, Shatin, Hong Kong*

**ONG KIM LIAN**
*Consultant in Accident and Emergency Medicine, Accident and Emergency Department, Prince of Wales Hospital, Shatin, Hong Kong*

and

**LAWRENCE TAN THUAN HENG**
*Senior Medical Officer, Department of Radiology, North District Hospital, Fanling, Hong Kong*

**OXFORD**
UNIVERSITY PRESS

# OXFORD
UNIVERSITY PRESS

Oxford University Press, Great Clarendon Street, Oxford OX2 6DP

Oxford University Press is a department of the University of Oxford
and furthers the University's aim of excellence in research, scholarship,
and education by publishing worldwide in

Oxford New York

Athens Auckland Bangkok Bogota Buenos Aires Calcutta
Cape Town Chennai Dar es Salaam Delhi Florence Hong Kong Istanbul
Karachi Kuala Lumpur Madrid Melbourne Mexico City Mumbai
Nairobi Paris São Paulo Singapore Taipei Tokyo Toronto Warsaw

and associated companies in Berlin Ibadan

Oxford is a trade mark of Oxford University Press

Published in the United States
by Oxford University Press, Inc., New York

British Library Cataloguing in Publication Data

Cocks, Robert.
Imaging in trauma / Robert Cocks, Ong Kim Lian, and Lawrence Tan Thuan Heng.
p.    cm.
Includes bibliographical references and index.
1. Diagnostic imaging.    2. Wounds and injuries—Diagnosis.
I. Lian, Ong Kim.    II. Heng, Lawrence Tan Thuan.    III. Title.
[DNLM: 1. Wounds and Injuries—diagnosis.    2. Diagnostic Imaging—methods.
3. Tomography, X-Ray Computed—methods.    WO 700 C666i   1999]
RC78.7.D53C62    1999    617.1′0754—dc21    99-16260
Library of Congress Cataloging in Publication Data

ISBN 0 19 262509 8

1 3 5 7 9 10 8 6 4 2

Typeset by Best-set Typesetter Ltd., Hong Kong
Printed in India by Thomson Press Ltd

# Preface

In recent years, trauma has been recognized as one of the most important healthcare issues still to be fully addressed. A new awareness of deficiencies in the clinical management of injured patients has led to an urgent reappraisal of procedures and training in many hospitals. At the same time, there has been a revolution in the field of radiology and diagnostic imaging. This handbook aims to bring together these parallel advances in order that imaging can be viewed as an integral part of clinical management.

The text promotes the safe and effective application of imaging techniques to patients who have been injured—to recommend techniques wherever they are known to be effective and to advise against their use where this would be inappropriate. The use of basic conventional radiology is most comprehensively covered, recognizing that some of the newer modalities, such as magnetic resonance imaging, will not be generally available for some years. The potential of newer techniques is discussed together with information about developments in computed radiography, ultrasound scanning, and computed tomography (CT) scanning.

It is, of course, important to consider not only the production of good images, but also how to help clinicians to order them appropriately and to interpret them. A full report from a trained radiologist may not be available immediately to junior medical staff trying to manage the patient in the Accident and Emergency (A&E) department. Therefore, advice about viewing images systematically is offered, together with hints on the pitfalls that might be faced. This advice is patient centred rather than image centred—an emphasis that makes the text different from others.

The book will be of assistance to all medical and nursing staff working in the speciality of accident and emergency medicine and also to those working in specialities that offer definitive care to injured patients. The production of informative images requires the efforts of nurses, doctors, radiographers, radiologists, and support staff, and all need to be familiar with their part in the process.

The contents of the book may also assist those wishing to study for higher examinations in accident and emergency medicine, surgery, and radiology, especially where the interpretation of images forms part of the examination.

*Hong Kong*
*August 1999*

R. A. C.
O. K. L.
L. T. T. H.

# Acknowledgements

We are most grateful to our patients for both the inspiration to prepare this book and also for the images contained within it.

Special thanks are owed to Mrs Ellen Chan, who has helped us to manage the main manuscript throughout, and has kept it tidy. We are also especially indebted to a member of our nursing staff, Ms Tan Chun Fung, who has skilfully prepared the line illustrations, and to Louise Johnson of the Medical Illustration Department of the former Salford Health Authority for drawing Fig. 4.3.

The Publishers would like to thank Dr Robin Illingworth for his valuable advice during the preparation of this book.

# Contents

## Part 4   Training, audit, and the future

## Appendices

# Introduction: the approach of this book

Most radiology textbooks will begin with an account of the physics of imaging and progress to descriptions of how to read films. This book takes a different approach—it starts with the physics of the accident and aims to promote an understanding of how the injuries might have taken place. By the time the reader gets to looking at the radiographs, he or she should have a mental image of what happened to the patient, and what to look for on the films.

The key to the approach is the *imaging plan*, a plan that every doctor dealing with the trauma patient can formulate on the basis of an understanding of the accident, and from results of the physical examination. The imaging plan may lead to an active decision *not* to do any investigations (as in the case of a clinically fractured coccyx in a teenage girl), or it may lead straight to a specialist investigation (for example, a preliminary CT scan rather than a skull X-ray in a head-injured patient who is in a coma).

An understanding of the mechanism of injury is vital in the diagnosis of injuries, and without it, failures of communication occur. Since trauma may not result in any accurate external physical signs of internal injury, the history is often by far the most important factor. Radiologists frequently complain of the lack of history given to them, and even very experienced ones may miss injuries if 'kept in the dark'. With over 200 bones in the human body, a radiologist can be forgiven for missing a fracture in a packet of films when the only history given is 'involved in RTA—multiple injuries'. Since trauma occurs at all hours of the day and night, A&E doctors frequently have to interpret the films alone. An understanding of what happened (and therefore what to look for) is crucial. Members of the ambulance crew are likely to know more about the mechanism of injury than anyone else, and the imaging plan therefore begins with information given by them.

The first part of the book describes the available techniques and the organization of imaging. The second part explores the effective clinical use of imaging techniques, and the third contains a systematic consideration of each part of the body. The final part discusses education, training, and audit, and some possibilities for the future use of trauma imaging.

# The imaging plan:
# key points

The planning of radiology and other forms of diagnostic imaging in trauma depends on:

- an understanding of the mechanism of injury, including secondary events;

- thorough physical examination;

- an understanding of the limitations and pitfalls of each investigation;

- the doctor's ability to communicate effectively with ambulance staff, nurses, radiographers, radiologists, and the on-take clinical teams.

# PART 1
# *The production and reporting of images*

# CHAPTER 1

# The techniques available

- Instant photography
- Conventional radiography
- Computed radiography
- Contrast radiography
- Computed tomography
- Ultrasonography
- Doppler imaging
- Angiography
- Radionuclide imaging
- Magnetic resonance imaging
- Bibliography

## INSTANT PHOTOGRAPHY

While not usually considered part of the imaging of a trauma patient, plain photography may provide very useful information.

Some ambulance services now carry instant cameras which are used to record information at the scene, including the position of a trapped patient and of vehicle damage. This information assists the Accident and Emergency (A&E) staff in gaining an impression of the mechanism of the accident, as may be seen from the example in Fig. 1.1.

A further benefit of instant photography is in the recording of the immediate appearance of a compound limb fracture. The wound can then be dressed and protected from contamination until the patient reaches the operating theatre. Restricted viewing has been proven to reduce the infection rate from 19.2 per cent to 4.3 per cent. An average of nine people may look at (and breathe over) a compound fracture between the accident scene and the operating theatre. Under Tscherne's regime, the wound was dressed at the scene and only exposed in theatre under full aseptic conditions (Tscherne 1983).

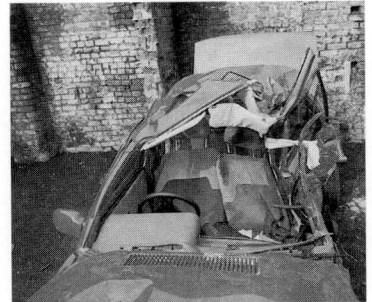

**Fig. 1.1** Instant photography: photograph taken by an ambulance crew at the accident scene.

A photographic record of wounds and injuries is often valuable for later medico-legal use. Many hospitals do not have the facilities to provide medical photography out of office hours, and the instant camera is valuable in filling this gap, although care is needed to achieve good results. All photography should form part of the patient's medical record and be subject to the patient's consent, if this can reasonably be obtained. The instant photographs must be dated and signed by the person taking them, and the patient's name and A&E number recorded on the back or foot of the image.

# CONVENTIONAL RADIOGRAPHY

Conventional radiography, a technique now over 100 years old, is still the main type of imaging in Accident and Emergency departments. The technique makes use of the fact that X-rays (generated by an X-ray tube, see Fig. 1.2) are absorbed to different degrees by different tissues, and that the portion that is not absorbed can be detected on a film or by another device.

It is important to advise the radiographer about the exact diagnostic purpose of the radiograph, since this may affect the current and voltage settings chosen for best results. This is particularly important in the imaging of foreign bodies, as will be seen later.

## Portable films

Portable (mobile) X-ray machines are commonly found in the operating theatres or resuscitation room in the Accident and Emergency department.

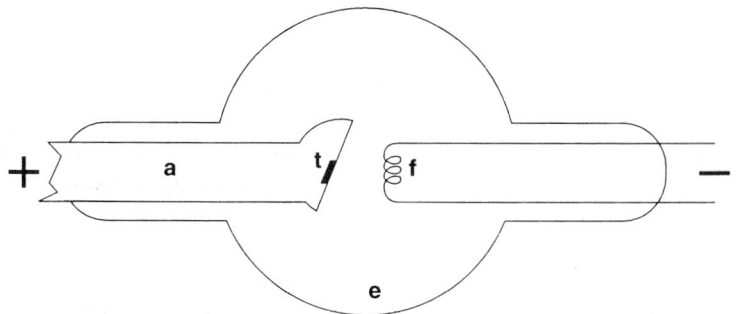

**Fig. 1.2** Major components of an X-ray tube: a, copper anode; e, vacuum envelope; f, heated tungsten filament; t, tungsten target.

Films taken using these portable machines have several limitations, which include limited exposure capabilities and underexposed films in very obese patients. Another potential pitfall lies in poor positioning of the patient on the resuscitation trolley, making reading of the films difficult due to artefacts and alteration of anatomical landmarks.

In most instances, a portable radiograph can provide enough crucial information to make critical clinical decisions, but overall, the quality of imaging is poorer than films taken in the radiology department.

# COMPUTED RADIOGRAPHY

An X-ray beam is generated using the same type of equipment as for conventional radiography, but instead of the conventional screen–film combination used to record the X-ray image, a photostimulable phosphor storage imaging plate is used. This imaging plate uses phosphors that act as radiation energy sensors to trap and store energy as a latent image.

To obtain the image, a laser scanner scans the imaging plate, resulting in the release of the stored energy as luminescence. This is then converted into digital signals, and using proprietary image-processing software, the digitized image signals then can be manipulated, transmitted, displayed, or stored, like any digital electronic data.

The processed digitized image can be stored in complete or compressed form on any electronic storage media, such as compact discs, or alternatively printed as hard-copy films.

# CONTRAST RADIOGRAPHY

## Contrast media

Contrast media are used widely with all imaging modalities to increase contrast between various tissues, to depict the hollow viscera, to study blood vessels and the flow within them, to assess organ function, and, on occasion, to facilitate interventional procedures.

## Barium sulphate

This inert material is used as a suspension in water, primarily to study the gastrointestinal tract. Double-contrast techniques using air or methylcellulose provide excellent studies of the mucosa in detail.

However, barium contrast is normally avoided in patients who are suspected of having bowel perforation.

## Water-soluble iodinated contrast media

Apart from their tissue-enhancing properties, these media can also be used to visualize blood vessels directly (angiography) or to opacify the urinary tract after being excreted by the kidneys. Water-soluble contrast material is used in routine radiography to demonstrate fistulas, sinuses, and perforations.

The use of newer (and relatively expensive) low osmolar or non-ionic contrast material can reduce the minor complications that commonly follow the injection of hypertonic iodine-containing contrast media. Some authors have reported reduced mortality rates from anaphylactic reactions with the use of non-ionic contrast media.

Recommended indications for the use of non-ionic contrast media in patients include:

(1) previous history of adverse reaction to iodinated contrast material;

(2) history of asthma or allergy;

(3) known cardiac dysfunction;

(4) generalized debilitation.

## Magnetic resonance imaging (MRI) contrast agents

MRI contrast agents are far safer than the compounds used in conventional radiography and computed tomography. They are usually chelates of gadolinium used as tissue-enhancing agents in order to produce effects similar to those of iodinated contrast media for computed tomography. Orally administered MRI contrast media for outlining the gastrointestinal tract are limited in their usefulness and are expensive.

# COMPUTED TOMOGRAPHY (CT)

CT uses X-rays generated in much the same way as for conventional radiography. However, instead of utilizing film or a fluorescent screen–film combination for image capture, a crystal or gas detector system of much greater sensitivity is used to generate digital information.

The X-ray tube and the detector rotate around the patient at the region of interest. Data collected is processed by computer to reconstruct a horizontal slice of the body comprised of small blocks of varying density. It is also possible to reconstruct three-dimensional images, a technique which is particularly useful for the face and spine, where the anatomy of fractures may be difficult to define. Unlike conventional radiography, CT can distinguish between various soft tissues and fluids (e.g. blood, cerebrospinal fluid). Intravenous contrast may be used to further improve diagnostic discrimination.

Recent developments have led to the introduction of spiral/helical CT. This offers continuous volume sampling, unlike the discrete cuts taken in conventional CT. The total scan times are shorter and, for example, the entire thorax can be scanned in a single breath-hold. Spiral CT has become the method of choice for paediatric patients and in situations where patients have to maintain an uncomfortable or awkward position.

# ULTRASONOGRAPHY

In diagnostic ultrasound examinations, echoes of very high frequency sound are used as a non-invasive means of imaging internal organs. To date, no harmful effects have been reported.

The transducer, containing a crystal that produces a predetermined ultrasound frequency, is placed in direct contact with the body area to be examined. The sound generated travels through the body, and at tissue interfaces echoes are reflected and picked up by the same crystal, which then converts them into electrical signals. These signals are processed and displayed as cross-sectional images on a cathode ray tube.

Ultrasonography is particularly useful in assessing density differences at fluid–solid interfaces, but is less useful where large differences exist (e.g. between gas and solid interfaces in the abdomen). Occasionally, better images may be obtained by interposing a fluid buffer, particularly where the body part has a complex shape, preventing good probe contact; for example, in the case of the ankle, a bag of saline may be used to create such a buffer.

The use of ultrasonography will be discussed in detail for each body region.

# DOPPLER IMAGING

Doppler imaging is a variation of ultrasonography used primarily to assess blood flow in vessels, and is particularly useful in detecting abnormal flow due to obstructions, for instance by injury or thrombosis. The technique employs sound waves aimed at a shallow angle towards the vessel in which blood is flowing. When the sound encounters moving blood, an echo is reflected at a different sound frequency. The difference in the frequencies is termed the Doppler shift.

Doppler ultrasound machines can produce pulsed and continuous signals. Pulsed Doppler gives the best results for detecting blood flow in an individual vessel, but continuous signals allow a flow picture to be generated of the whole image. Flow is revealed in real time within the selected region of interest. When different frequencies are displayed as different colours, a colour-flow Doppler image is generated. Generally, the colours are typically assigned as red and blue. Paler hues of the same colours are often assigned to higher Doppler shifts.

# ANGIOGRAPHY

Urgent diagnostic angiography is seldom performed in the Accident and Emergency department, but the use of this modality in appropriate cases may save limbs and lives. Patients in urgent need of this investigation are those requiring diagnostic decisions on the adequacy of limb circulation and those who may require urgent surgical intervention to repair major vascular structures.

An angiogram is an X-ray examination of blood vessels using iodinated contrast medium. The examination demonstrates not only the anatomy of both arteries and veins, but also the location of bleeding points as extravasation of contrast medium. To demonstrate a bleed, an ongoing blood loss of at least 0.5–0.6 ml/min must be present.

# RADIONUCLIDE IMAGING

The type of radionuclide imaging that can be performed depends on the availability of specific radiopharmaceuticals. The pharmaceutical component concentrates selectively in specific parts of the body and the attached radioactive isotopes emit gamma rays as they decay. These rays are detected by a scintillation counter, the signals being processed and recorded as a print-out of dots which vary in number depending on the intensity of radiation. Some uses include establishing the presence of gastrointestinal bleeding, assessing patency of ventriculoperitoneal (VP) shunts, and in demonstrating subtle fractures that are not easily seen on conventional radiography.

When available, nuclear medicine scans may have a role in the following areas:

1. Non-accidental injuries: rib and physeal fractures may be subtle or invisible on a radiograph. Nuclear medicine bone scans can often demonstrate such subtle fractures.

2. The diagnosis of difficult fractures (e.g. scaphoid): if the diagnosis can be established, appropriate treatment can be given earlier, often without the need to wait for a 10-day repeat radiograph to determine the presence of a scaphoid fracture.

3. Gastrointestinal tract bleeding: nuclear medicine scanning is more sensitive than angiography in locating the source of bleeding. If the scan is positive, it can then help to guide the subsequent angiogram for therapeutic embolization. The rate of bleeding must be at least 0.5–1 ml/min for angiographic detection, while a bleeding rate of 0.1–0.2 ml/min is often positive on a radionuclide scan.

# MAGNETIC RESONANCE IMAGING (MRI)

MRI is an imaging technique that utilizes radio pulses of a specific frequency to 'excite' molecules in the body, releasing energy that can be detected and processed into images. The region of interest is placed within a powerful magnet. No ionizing radiation is used, but care must be taken to avoid imaging patients with cardiac pacemakers or intracranial ferromagnetic aneurysm clips, and orthopaedic metal plates or prostheses, which may loosen.

The use of MRI in the Accident and Emergency department is currently limited because it is expensive and because of the length of time required to complete the examination. Currently, MRI is considered particularly useful in the assessment of skeletal trauma, especially that of the spine. MRI is a rapidly developing imaging technique and the technology is constantly being improved and costs reduced, and thus it is likely to become more readily available for routine trauma imaging in the future.

# BIBLIOGRAPHY

Ballinger PW. Merrill's Atlas of Radiographic Positions and Radiologic Procedures, 8th edn. Missouri: Mosby, 1995; 3:43–320.

Ben Menachem Y. Imaging techniques in trauma. In: Maull KL, ed. Advances in Trauma and Critical Care. Chicago: Mosby, 1992; 7:191–217.

Chapman S, Nakielny R. A Guide to Radiological Procedures, 3rd edn. Baillière Tindall: WB Saunders, 1993.

Feliciano DV. Diagnostic modalities in abdominal trauma: peritoneal lavage, ultrasonography, computed tomography scanning and arteriography. Surg Clin North Am 1991; 71:241.

Leutz KA, Mckenny MG, Nunez DB, *et al*. Evaluating blunt abdominal trauma: role of ultrasonogrphy. J Ultrasound Med 1996; 15:447.

Tscherne H. Management of wounds in fractures with soft tissue injuries Z Kinderchir 1983; 38(1):34–9.

# CHAPTER 2

# The organization and logistics of imaging in the Accident and Emergency department

- Facilities necessary: location
- The ordering of imaging
- Staffing considerations
- Radiation protection
- Reference

## FACILITIES NECESSARY: LOCATION

All Accident and Emergency departments offering an unrestricted service must have radiology facilities available 24 hours each day, and the support staff to run them. While this is usually taken to mean availability of plain X-ray facilities, it is desirable that ultrasonography, angiography, and CT scanning should also be readily available to avoid unnecessary secondary transfers.

For the most seriously ill and injured patients, radiology is needed within the resuscitation room. The gold standard for resuscitation room facilities must be the gantry-mounted X-ray tube, but equally good-quality radiography can also be ensured by replicating full resuscitation room facilities in a dedicated A&E X-ray room.

In the majority of A&E departments, the three baseline films recommended by the Advanced Trauma Life Support® guidelines are taken using a mobile X-ray machine. The quality of such films is good enough to detect major abnormalities of bony structures and alignment, but may not be adequate to rule out more subtle changes. Generally, detailed radiology of the skull, spine, and limbs should be deferred until the patient is stable enough to benefit from the more reliable fixed equipment in the X-ray room.

In general, the fixed radiology facilities available to the Accident and Emergency department should be located either within the department or directly adjacent to it, on the same floor. Any facilities located outside the department have two drawbacks—first, the patient is no longer close to the resuscitation facilities and expertise of the A&E department, and, secondly, trained A&E nursing staff accompanying the patient are taken away from the A&E department. A survey in one A&E department, with radiology facilities on the floor above, showed that an average of 40 hours per week of nursing staff time was spent accompanying patients for X-rays.

Any X-ray rooms used for emergency patients which are not located within the A&E department must be equipped with at least basic resuscitation equipment and drugs, the location and layout of which should be known to all radiographers and accompanying nursing and medical staff. The checking and restocking of these facilities is an important task, which could be undertaken by A&E department staff.

Unlike the larger North American emergency rooms, few A&E departments in the United Kingdom have their own CT scanning facilities. However, most district general hospitals now have a CT scanner that can be used for the benefit of trauma patients, although not all are available on a 24-hour service basis.

Hospitals that provide a service for vascular trauma must also have 24-hour availability of angiography, both for prompt initial investigation and for on-table imaging during corrective surgery.

In the UK, magnetic resonance imaging is rarely available in the acute phase of trauma management, but in the future this may change.

# ORDERING OF IMAGING

In the view of the Royal College of Radiologists, the X-ray request form is analogous to a request for a clinical consultation, 'In most situations the request is entirely appropriate. In some cases the best examination for resolving the problem may be a different imaging modality. Occasionally the request itself may not be appropriate' (Royal College of Radiologists 1993).

Communication with radiographers and radiologists is crucial to the success of the imaging plan. The requesting clinician must have a clear idea of why he or she is ordering a particular examination, and communicate this clearly to the radiology staff. If these conditions are not satisfied, the potential for errors at each step along the way is magnified. For example, if the clinician is interested in detecting a foreign body retained in the tissues and does not communicate this, the radiographer may not be able to choose the appropriate exposure that would offer the greatest chance of detection.

Poor communication can also compromise the effectiveness of the 'safety net' system (see Chapter 3). Junior medical staff in the A&E department may develop a tendency to provide skimpy details on the X-ray request form because they know that they themselves will be interpreting the radiograph ('why bother writing lots when I know what I'm looking for?'). However, if they happen to miss an abnormality, the chances of the radiologist spotting it when checking the films later are reduced, because of the poor history given.

The imaging request form must contain accurate patient details. If a patient is admitted unconscious and cannot be identified, their sex and unique A&E number must be given as a minimum on the form. An estimated age is also helpful. Adopting a convention of the sort of format 'Unknown male 1, A&E No. 635128H, approx. 50 years' might be an effective way to preventing confusion in a multiple casualty road accident between, for example, a father and son or grandson. Ethnic identification codes, as used by the police, are not well understood by hospital staff and may be less useful in multiple casualty incidents (all of the members of a family in one vehicle may share the same ethnic code).

The age of the patient (even approximate) is important in interpreting the radiographs—epiphyses in the child, osteophytes and osteoporosis in later life are features that require a knowledge of age to place them in the correct context in a radiologist's report.

The doctor ordering radiology for trauma patients must balance the benefits of the study against the risks. Females of childbearing age are a particular group who require careful consideration. The clinician has a responsibility to enquire about the possibility of pregnancy and to inform the radiology department before investigations are done. In patients with major trauma, the benefits of investigation will almost always outweigh the risks, even in the presence of a pregnancy. There may be some potential for shielding the abdomen and genital area if the radiology department is told in advance, particularly while skull, cervical spine, chest, and extremity X-rays are being performed. In pregnant patients with less serious trauma, radiology between the diaphragm and knees should be avoided unless essential for overriding clinical reasons. A decision may need to be made by a senior clinician in these cases.

The 'clinical details' section on the request form should always be completed as fully as possible. The circumstances of the trauma (e.g. 'road traffic accident') need to be given, followed by the mechanism (e.g. 'front seat passenger—side impact', etc.). The specific examination findings and suspected injuries should then be given, as well as details of any complicating medical conditions.

Full discussion of the indications for different investigations will follow in Part 2, but it is worth considering briefly the medico-legal aspects of ordering radiology. Doctors may sometimes feel that they must order an radiograph to avoid criticism or litigation. This feeling may be reinforced by the patient demanding an X-ray, even when the doctor feels that none is necessary.

*The decision to order any form of imaging must be based on clinical considerations alone.*

Investigations ordered for any other reason are difficult to justify and represent unnecessary irradiation of the patient. The imaging plan is an effective way of justifying any decision to order, or not order, an investigation. Careful thoughts, recorded in the case notes and on the request form, offer more legal defence than poorly written notes and a cursory look at a radiograph taken as a 'safety shot'.

# STAFFING CONSIDERATIONS: PATIENT DEPENDENCIES

Many imaging procedures in trauma are labour-intensive and require movement of the patient to achieve optimal results. Sufficient skilled staff must be available to produce the right conditions—even if this means a temporary reduction in other less urgent activity in the A&E department.

The level of attention the patient requires is governed by his or her triage category, both clinically and radiologically. Patients with major trauma are placed in category 1—indicating that immediate attention is required, as a threat to their life or health would occur in the event of delay. Implicit in this 'immediate' categorization is the requirement for the patient to be managed and accompanied by staff possessing a high level of skill. This requirement extends to the clinical management of the patient during more complex imaging (e.g. CT scanning) and during transport to and from it. It may happen that the A&E staffing levels would be seriously depleted by this degree of commitment, and each department needs to negotiate effective arrangements with other specialties (such as anaesthesia, the intensive care unit (ICU), and surgery) to provide medical and nursing staff back-up.

While all radiographers possess a broad range of skills, many A&E departments have found that extra benefits follow from the appointment of dedicated A&E radiography staff. These benefits tend to derive from the ability of all groups of staff to work together as members of a familiar team, who concentrate on the common purpose of dealing with emergency patients and the unique challenges they present.

# RADIATION PROTECTION

When requesting any radiological investigation, the clinician must bear in mind that all X-rays are potentially carcinogenic and terato-genic. Adequate radiation protection should be employed for the patient and for the attending healthcare staff.

## Female patients of reproductive age

Medical staff should check the menstrual history in patients of child-bearing age who need radiography of any body area. The examination should preferably be postponed if the last menstrual period began more than 28 days previously, unless the patient can be sure that there is no risk of pregnancy. This '28-day rule' has replaced the 10-day rule previously recommended by the Royal College of Radiologists.

## The pregnant patient

Irradiation of any area from the diaphragm to the knees should be avoided, especially in the first trimester, unless there are overriding clinical considerations.

## Staff

Continuous fluoroscopy screening is rarely employed in A&E depart-ments, total doses of radiation to individual non-radiography staff members should be low, and personal dosimeters are probably unnec-essary. Whenever X-rays are being used in the resuscitation room, CT room, or theatre, staff remaining with the patient should wear lead aprons, which reduce scattered radiation exposure by a factor of 30.

# REFERENCE

Royal College of Radiologists Making the best use of a department of clinical radiology—guidelines for doctors. 4th. edition, 1998. Royal College of Radiologists, London.

# CHAPTER 3

# *The reporting of images and safety-net systems*

- Radiographer reporting: the red dot system
- Interpretation by the requesting clinician
- Hot reporting by a radiologist
- Cold reporting; safety nets; recall

## RADIOGRAPHER REPORTING: THE RED DOT SYSTEM

Assessing the quality of an image is part of every radiographer's job. During the course of this checking, their trained eyes may spot an abnormality that a junior A&E doctor might miss. Although radiographers are not able to report formally on images in detail, the benefit of their expertise in locating subtle abnormalities should not be lost. One way of 'flagging' an abnormal film for the attention of the A&E doctor is for a red dot to be placed on the film as a caution marker. Even if the doctor cannot see what is wrong, he or she can then discuss the film with the radiographer, and a radiologist if necessary.

This system offers considerable opportunity for staff education and training by means of a regular audit process.

## INTERPRETATION BY THE REQUESTING CLINICIAN

The majority of all A&E images taken are initially interpreted by the doctor who requested them in the first instance. In some ways, this doctor has the best opportunity of all to home in on a possible abnormality, and has the advantage of having both the image and the patient to compare (unlike the radiologist later on). For this reason it is undesirable that junior medical staff (or even senior ones!) should interpret radiographs for each other in isolation. This bad practice happens particularly often at the end of an A&E shift, when radiographs may be ordered before one doctor goes off duty, which are then seen by another doctor. The second doctor placed in this position should always make a brief clinical examination of the injured part before looking at the images. Many avoidable mistakes happen for lack of doing this.

All medical staff who are expected to interpret their own images must receive some training when they join the A&E service, and this topic is covered in more detail in Part 4. It is unreasonable to expect an A&E senior house officer to develop very detailed interpretation skills, and the training will inevitably concentrate on the recognition of patterns and common abnormalities.

## HOT REPORTING BY THE RADIOLOGIST

Increasingly, radiology departments offer a 'hot reporting' system in which images are examined and reported by a radiologist soon after being taken. If a well-run system is in place, only brief delays occur, which are far outweighed by the additional benefit to the patient of an expert opinion. However, in very busy departments, pressure of such work can lead to unacceptable delays, particularly if images have to be transported some distance from the A&E X-ray room to the radiology department. Delays may also occur if the radiology facilities are overloaded by other clinical activity in progress—a fracture clinic for instance.

The best hot-reporting systems include the possibility for the referring clinician to be present during the reporting of the film. Very few hospitals have 24-hour hot reporting, but the teaching value of even a limited system, in which both radiologist and clinician participate, can be invaluable preparation for the times when the clinician must cope on his or her own.

Radiologists have a good knowledge of normal variants and age-related normal anatomy, and the hot-reporting system may help reduce false-positive diagnoses as well as increasing the pick-up rate for real abnormalities. A significant proportion of imaging requests may be asking for the wrong investigation—the radiologist can readily advise on the optimal methods of additional imaging for a particular condition.

## COLD REPORTING; SAFETY NETS; RECALL

Even with the best intentions, the misdiagnosis rate on A&E radiographs runs at between 1 and 5 per cent. It is therefore very important that all images taken of patients in the Accident and Emergency department should be reported on by a radiologist as soon as possible after the patient's attendance. A further, related consideration is that images taken on A&E patients who are subsequently admitted to hospital may also show unrecognized abnormalities— these images too must be subject to early reporting.

Ideally, images need to be reported within 24 hours of the patient's attendance or admission. This will allow for serious abnormalities (e.g. a missed skull fracture, pneumothorax, or pneumoperitoneum) to be recognized and the patient recalled immediately. However, this goal is rarely achieved at weekends in most hospitals, due to staffing considerations. Most simple limb fractures can withstand a delay of 3–4 days before treatment, but a legal question then arises concerning compensation for 'unnecessary pain and suffering' experienced by the patient in the meantime. Reporting within 24 hours must remain the standard for good practice.

A second element in the safety net is the presence of a mechanism for reacting to the discovery of an abnormality on cold reporting. The radiologist must be able to contact a senior A&E clinician with reasonable ease, and that clinician then needs to make a judgement regarding the recall of the patient. This sort of situation really underscores the need for the adequate collection of patient information (the correct address, telephone number, name of GP, etc.). The first action will be to attempt contact with the patient by telephone. If this is not possible, an attempt is made to contact the GP, who might then visit the patient. In really serious cases, where these two moves have failed, the A&E clinician might consider sending an appropriate member of the A&E staff to the patient's address by police or ambulance transport, to look for them and assure their safety. In less serious cases, where all attempts at contact have failed, a recall letter might be sent. In any event, the system in the Accident and Emergency department must be clear, and the action taken should be recorded in the clinical notes. Persistent attempts may be needed.

The absence of an adequate safety-net system may be more damning in the courts than the fact that a misdiagnosis has occurred. As with intubation of the oesophagus, the crime is not in doing it, but in failing to recognize that it might have occurred and acting appropriately. A mistake or misdiagnosis is not in itself indicative of negligence (if reasonable care can be shown to have been taken).

# PART 2
## *The clinical use of imaging*

# CHAPTER 4

# General principles of imaging in the trauma patient

........................................................................................................................................................................................................................

- Making an imaging plan
- How force translates into injury: common patterns
- Patterns of injury

## MAKING AN IMAGING PLAN

The approach to any trauma patient must be uniform. Clinical procedures are described in more detail in Chapter 5.

The first aim is to detect and treat life-threatening injuries and physiological derangements (primary survey), followed by stabilizing measures, followed by a detailed examination from top to toe (secondary survey). After completing the initial assessment, work through the following mental checklist:

1.  Do I understand what happened? If the patient does not know or is unable to give details, have I spoken to the ambulance crew, traffic police, relatives, or other eye witnesses who might be in the department, and who might be leaving soon? If I do not have a clear idea of what occurred, is there anyone I can contact to find out for me?

2.  Have I completed a thorough physical examination as part of the secondary survey, and in detail wherever I have found an injury? Do these findings tie up with my understanding of the injury mechanism?

3.  For every injured part of the body, what investigation could help me establish the nature and extent of the injury? From the mechanism, what would I *expect* to find? If I don't find it, does the investigation reliably rule out the injury? Is there another investigation that might help, and do I need to seek the advice of a radiologist?

4.  Is the patient stable enough to leave the A&E department for any special investigation I have considered? Who needs to accompany the patient during the investigation, and what equipment, blood, and drugs will be required to make the patient safe? What is the worst that could happen, and how should it be handled? Does the need for the investigation outweigh the risk?

5.  Who do I need to communicate with in order to make the imaging process work smoothly? Are porters available, nursing staff and radiographers briefed, and are they all ready at the same time? If I am not staying with the patient, who is in charge, and do they understand my plan?

If this approach is taken, the process of obtaining images will be smooth and as safe as possible.

## HOW FORCE TRANSLATES INTO INJURY: COMMON PATTERNS

### Bone

Forces causing injury to the bones may be direct or indirect. An example of an accident involving direct force would be the impact of a car bumper with the lower leg, causing injury to the tibia. Indirect injury to the same bone might occur when a skier loses control, causing torsional force to be applied to the tibia. In each case, the radiological appearance can be predicted from the mechanism history. Direct forces tend to produce transverse, comminuted fractures which are often also compound—air may be seen in the subcutaneous tissues or around the bone fragments. Torsion of the bone is more likely to produce a spiral or oblique fracture, less commonly compound.

However, direct trauma may cause effects remote from the point of application of the force, especially in the case of rings or spheres of bone (e.g. pelvis, skull). Direct trauma to one part of the circle may not produce fractures at that precise site, but distortion of the circle may produce a break at its weakest point.

Different degrees of concentration of a direct force onto the bone may produce different effects. Consider, for instance, a small pebble falling from a cliff and striking the head of a person on the beach below. The pebble is of small mass but high velocity. The absorption of the pebble's kinetic energy (half of its mass times the square of its velocity) over a small area of the person's skull is likely to produce a localized, compound fracture, perhaps with some depression of bone fragments into the cranial cavity. Now consider a grapefruit-sized rock, much heavier but falling from a lesser height, with the same kinetic energy as the pebble. This rock would be likely to cause a more diffuse injury—perhaps a 'pond' fracture where the skull breaks at the point of maximum convexity and also more remotely at the edges of the area to which force is applied.

## Bones and tendons

In response to loss of balance or sudden movement of a joint, sudden reflex muscle contractions may occur which result in abnormal loading of the tendons beyond their tolerance. A common example of this is the sudden contraction of peroneus brevis during an inversion injury to the ankle when a person stumbles and loses their balance. The contraction is sometimes forceful enough to rip off the styloid of the fifth metatarsal bone, leaving a clear gap visible on radiography.

Similar appearances may be seen at other sites of insertion of tendon into bone, for example the insertion of the extensor mechanism of a finger into the distal phalanx. Occasionally, the radiological appearances are barely visible, with only a few tiny flecks of bone to mark the end of the avulsed extensor tendon.

## Bones and ligaments

The skeleton is held together by ligaments, with varying degrees of movement possible at the fibrous, cartilaginous, and synovial joints. When the maximum range of movement at a particular joint in any direction is exceeded, the resulting overtension of the ligament results in either tearing of the ligament (partially or completely) or the ligament pulling away from the bone to which it is attached. As with tendons, discussed previously, pieces of bone may be avulsed as well and be visible on radiographs.

The ankle is one of the most commonly injured joints, inversion being the commonest mechanism. When the foot inverts, the lateral collateral ligament of the ankle (made up of three portions) is stretched. This may result in injury to the ligament, ranging from minor damage ('sprain') to complete rupture. One radiographic sign may be partial separation of the edge of the fibular malleolus (with small flecks of bone which can be seen adjacent to the edge). If the ligament remains intact, a larger part of the malleolus may be avulsed.

Similar effects may be seen at many other sites in the body (e.g. avulsion of parts of the anterior cervical vertebral bodies in hyperextension injuries).

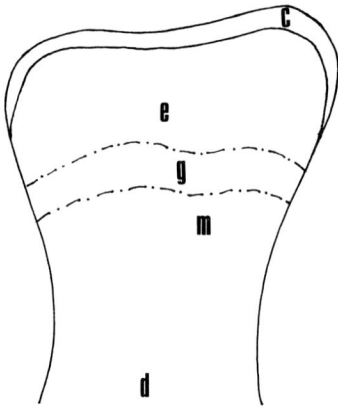

**Fig. 4.1** Immature skeleton: normal physis in long bone. c, Cartilage cap; d, diaphysis (shaft); e, epiphysis; g, growth plate; m, metaphysis.

## Bones and their epiphyses

Bones grow at their extremities by means of epiphyseal (growth) plates, the pattern of which varies depending on the shape of the bone. For long bones, the main shaft is termed the diaphysis, and this ossifies first from a primary ossification centre. At each end are the epiphyses and their growth plates (sometimes multiple) which eventually fuse with the diaphysis as secondary ossification centres (see Fig. 4.1).

Epiphyseal injuries are covered in more detail in Chapter 16.

## Solid organs

Modern imaging techniques offer the possibility of demonstrating damage to tissues other than bones.

Solid organs (e.g. liver, spleen, and brain) are most commonly affected by direct trauma. Damage to them can be predicted from the mechanism of the injury—severe deceleration may cause the organ to deform against a bony structure (e.g. the skull vault or the inner ribcage), or an external force may strike the stationary organ.

Secondary effects of injury may cause further damage to solid organs. An example of this would be the formation of an intracranial haematoma, which may enlarge and compress the brain, causing structural distortion and ischaemia.

In most cases, it is not possible to produce reliably good images of solid organs using standard conventional radiography. The possible exception to this is in the case of the lung, in which there are sharp solid–liquid–air interfaces with little surrounding tissue to obscure the view. More usually, contrast radiography, ultrasound, computed tomography (CT), and magnetic resonance imaging (MRI) offer more information, and these will be discussed in detail for each body region.

## Hollow organs

Hollow organs are most susceptible to direct blunt or penetrating mechanical trauma. Portions of the bowel that contain gas and semi-solids (e.g. the small intestine) are unlikely to be ruptured by diffuse blunt injury; more concentrated trauma is usually involved. An example would be the sort of insult caused by an incorrectly adjusted seat-belt lap strap, which in a frontal collision may tighten against the abdomen, causing a sudden rise in internal hydrostatic pressure in a loop of bowel. Solid-filled portions of bowel (e.g. the colon) are susceptible to direct trauma, particularly where they are fixed to the posterior abdominal wall. Penetrating injury may result in perforation of any hollow organ.

Imaging of the actual damage to hollow organs is difficult and usually relies on contrast studies, but the secondary effects of rupture (leakage of air or fluid) may be easier to locate. Plain erect chest X-rays are useful to detect air under the diaphragm, but may be impossible to obtain in many multiple trauma patients, due to unconsciousness or because spinal injury cannot be excluded. Ultrasonography may detect fluid collections from rupture of the bladder or bowel, as may CT scanning. Contrast studies may be able to identify precisely the site of leakage in hollow organs.

## The vascular tree

The heart and vascular structures are particularly susceptible to penetrating trauma, but may also be damaged by indirect mechanisms. For example, a workman falling from a height and landing on his feet sustains a vertical deceleration. The heart has momentum and continues to move downwards when the body comes to a halt, placing stress on the arch of the aorta. The aorta may be torn at the arch either completely or partially, the mortality initially depending on whether the rupture is contained or free. Any leakage of blood resulting from an aortic tear may be seen on appropriate images. Significant free haemorrhage into the chest cavity will be visible on chest X-ray. If the leak is contained within an intact mediastinum, the blood may widen the mediastinum and also track over the domes of the pleura, creating an apical pleural cap. The aortic knuckle is often obscured.

Fractures and dislocation of bones may compress, distort, or tear blood vessels at many sites in the body. A thorough clinical examination is a prerequisite for the complete imaging plan, in order to detect vascular deficiencies distal to the obvious site of injury. In particular, peripheral pulses should be marked with a pen and observed regularly.

Ultrasonography may detect haematoma resulting from vascular disruption, but most injuries require the use of contrast angiography to achieve detailed site location.

## PATTERNS OF INJURY

All injuries are caused by a transfer of energy to the body. If the mechanism of that transfer can be understood, then the injuries can be predicted (or at least suspected). Unfortunately, physical examination may not always give much of a clue to underlying injuries.

Consider for instance an assault victim who has received a hard blow to the upper abdomen from the assailant's knee. Such a patient is unlikely to have any mark on the abdomen at all. However, the likelihood of solid organ injury (particularly to the liver) is significant—the patient may be unconscious and shocked and may not even show abdominal guarding or rigidity.

While a clear history may not always be available, the following paragraphs include some aspects to consider.

## Falls

Falls are amongst the most common causes of trauma. Many injuries in adults are due to falling over from the standing position (an event commonly assisted by alcohol). In children, a fall from standing rarely causes serious injury, and most cases coming to A&E have fallen from furniture or stairs or while running.

Falls from a height produce variable injuries, depending on the position of the body on impact. The potential energy of the body falling from a height (and therefore the injury potential) is calculated by the formula:

$$\text{potential energy} = \textit{m}\text{ass (kg)} \times \text{acceleration due to } \textit{g}\text{ravity (g)} \times \textit{h}\text{eight (m).}$$

The height element reduces to zero by the time the person strikes the ground, and by this time the potential energy has been transformed into kinetic energy of equal magnitude (less a small portion converted into heat by friction with the air on the way down). At the moment of impact, the kinetic energy is converted into mechanical energy, expended in causing the injuries.

We can compare the equivalence of falls and vehicular crashes using the above formula. For a 70 kg body, a dead-stop frontal impact in a vehicle travelling at 22 mph is equivalent to a fall of 5 m. However, doubling the speed of the crash to 44 mph equates to a fall of 20 m, a fourfold increase.

Some injury patterns emerge:

1. Falls directly onto the feet produce a well-defined range of injuries. Commonly, the impact on the heels produces calcaneal fractures. The next stage depends on whether the patient remains upright. If one ankle inverts, the body may fall sideways, resulting in subsequent injuries more characteristic of a fall onto the side. If the body remains upright, force is transmitted axially up the legs. The next points of weakness occur at the tibial plateaux, which may fracture under loading from the more massive femoral condyles. Higher up, forces have to change direction at the angular neck of the femur, possibly resulting in unilateral or bilateral hip fractures. If the femoral

necks remain intact, one or rarely both femoral heads may be driven through the acetabulum as a central dislocation (Fig. 4.2).

Further shifting of the line of force then takes place between the pelvis and sacrum to the spine in the midline, leading to shearing stresses and possible pelvic disruption through the symphysis pubis and sacroiliac joints (several variations are possible). Compressive forces on the spine may cause burst fractures of the vertebral bodies in any location up to the C1 ring and the skull base. If bending stresses on the spine also accompany compression, fractures are particularly common at the thoracolumbar junction but may occur anywhere along the spine.

While the loading is transmitted upwards from the impact of the feet with the floor, the internal organs continue to travel downwards. A faecally loaded colon may tear away from its mesentery, and the liver may disrupt structures joined to it (inferior vena cava (IVC), diaphragm, and peritoneal folds). As discussed earlier, downward motion of the heart may lead to tearing of the aorta.

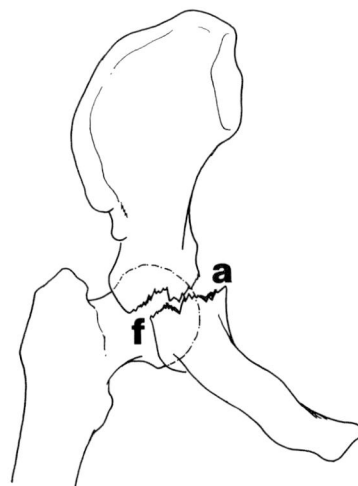

**Fig. 4.2** Hip: frontal view: a, acetabulum fracture; f, femoral head and neck intact.

2. Falls onto the side produce a pattern of injuries resulting from direct trauma and from deceleration of organs and their supports. Injuries to the pelvis and shoulder girdle are common, due to the protrusion of these areas. Serious injuries to the side of the head may occur, affecting vital brain areas more commonly than anterior or posterior impacts. In impacts with water resulting from falls from a great height (e.g. from the Golden Gate Bridge), patients entering the water on their side tend to have a worse outcome than those entering head or feet first.

## Pedestrian versus vehicle accidents

Unsurprisingly, a contact between a moving vehicle and a pedestrian has an unequal outcome—in fatal pedestrian versus car accidents in the UK in 1992, 97 per cent of those killed were pedestrians and only 3 per cent were vehicle occupants.

The pattern of injuries sustained depends on the type of vehicle and the direction and speed of impact. Impacts occur most commonly with the front of the vehicle hitting a pedestrian from the side. The sequence of events is an initial contact of the vehicle bumper with the patient's leg, usually at upper tibia/knee level. If a tibial fracture does not occur immediately, severe stresses are placed on the medial collateral ligament of the knee as a result of varus movement. Crushing of the lateral meniscus and lateral tibial plateau may occur before the cruciate ligaments are disrupted.

The weight of the body keeps the feet on the ground at this stage, but the body and legs may be displaced, causing injuries at or around the ankle. The body then leaves the ground and the hip and pelvis strike the leading edge of the bonnet. The upper body is then displaced sideways, the head hitting the windscreen or screen wiper hubs. In high-velocity accidents, the body may continue to travel over the roof of the car, with secondary injuries occurring when the victim hits the ground. If the body has been struck obliquely, the victim may be thrown sideways from the bonnet, into the path of other vehicles.

## Motorcycle accidents

Although motorcyclists enjoy better all-round vision than most vehicle drivers, they are more vulnerable in an impact. Although compulsory wearing of crash helmets has reduced the incidence of serious head injuries, other effective crash protection measures, such as leg protection, have not proved to be popular with manufacturers or motorcyclists. Common causes of accidents include loss of control of the machine in adverse weather conditions, collision with the back or front of cars and with cars emerging from side roads in front of riders. Lower-limb and pelvic injuries are common in primary motorcycle–vehicle impacts, and shoulder and head injuries in the secondary impact with the top of the vehicle or the ground. In free falls with no collision, extensive abrasions are commonly found due to friction against the road surface.

If the motorcycle collides at a shallow angle parallel with the side of a car or van, the leg involved in the impact may be forcibly abducted as the motorcycle continues to move down the side of the vehicle. This may result in closed pelvic disruption, and in rare cases a complete avulsion of the leg and hemipelvis occurs. Closed disruption of the pelvis (either anterior fracture with disrupted sacroiliac (SI) joint or symphysis disruption with disrupted SI joint) may not be obvious immediately on examination, and therefore radiology of the pelvis with an SI joint view is mandatory with this injury mechanism.

## Vehicle occupant injuries

Many design features of modern cars are intended to minimize injuries to the occupants in the event of an impact. Severe injuries to the chest were once common as a result of impact with a rigid steering column. In frontal impacts, the column would frequently be pushed upwards towards the driver, impaling the chest. Modern vehicles have steering columns which are discontinuous or which dislocate or fold up under impact conditions—features that have reduced the number of fatal injuries. The compulsory introduction of seat belts for front and rear occupants has similarly reduced mortality and has changed injury patterns significantly.

## Frontal impacts

Head-on or offset frontal impacts result in sudden deceleration of the vehicle, while the momentum of the occupants carries them forwards. A driver not wearing a seat belt will be projected forwards, striking his or her knees against the underside of the dashboard, chest against the steering wheel, and head against the windscreen as the body rises out of the seat. Prior to the impact, the driver may have attempted to brake hard. At impact, the right foot may be thrust between the pedals (foot pedal entrapment) and as the body moves forward, the tibia rotates in relation to the fixed foot, causing either malleolar injuries or a spiral fracture of the tibia. If parts of the engine are forced backwards into the footwell, this intrusion may also result in injury.

Impact of the knees against the dashboard may cause closed or compound injuries to the patella but also axial force is transmitted along the rigid strut formed by the femur. The hip joint is least stable in flexion—just the position in which the car driver is sitting—and the impact may therefore cause posterior dislocation of one or both hip joints.

If the driver is wearing a seat belt, the tension in the belt after the initial uptake of slack restrains forward movement. However, small drivers who sit close to the steering wheel may still sustain injuries to their chest or epigastrium. Although the body is restrained, the

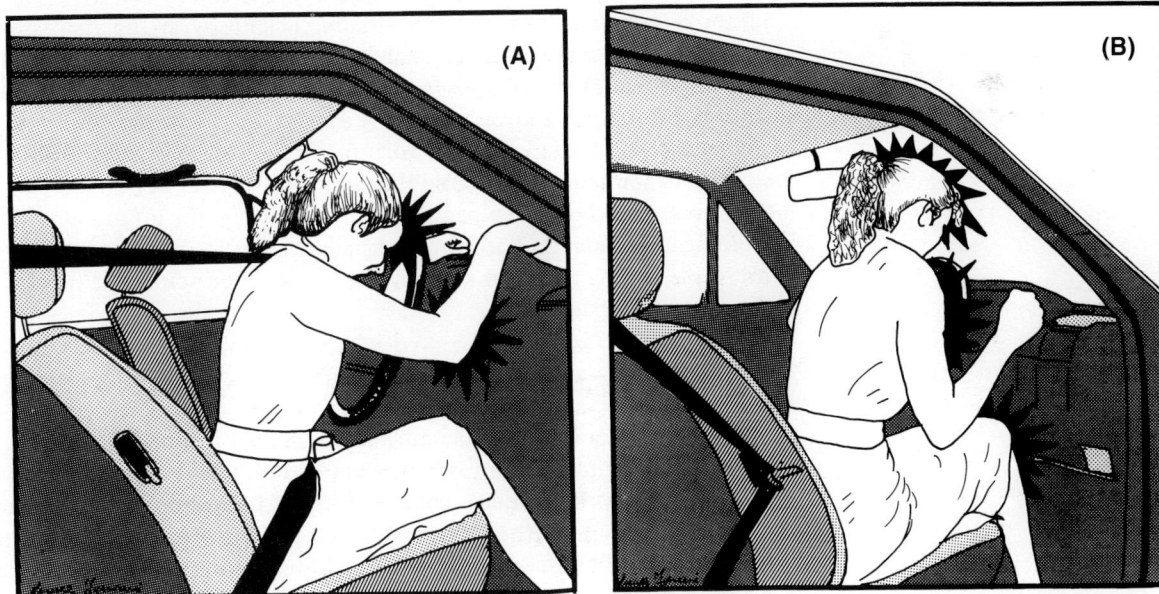

**Fig. 4.3** Patterns of injury: driver (A) with and (B) without seat-belt protection. Reconstruction of two actual cases.

relatively heavy head is free to move and continues to move forwards, forcibly flexing the neck. The head commonly strikes the top of the steering wheel even in restrained drivers, although head injuries are usually less severe than for the unrestrained driver. The introduction of air-bags in some vehicles has reduced the danger of steering wheel head trauma for both restrained and unrestrained drivers.

The seat belts themselves may cause injury. A driver's belt runs over the right clavicle, sternum, and left lower ribs. Heavy impact can cause fractures in any of these three areas, although myocardial contusion occurs less frequently with sternal fractures in belted drivers. The energy of impact is dissipated over about 300 cm$^2$ of belt area, only 10 per cent of which overlies the heart, as opposed to 100 cm$^2$ of steering-wheel hub, most of which overlies the heart. The force applied is a more gradual bending stress on the sternum rather than a sudden impact stress.

The lap part of the seat belt may cause injury to the bladder or pregnant uterus and, if poorly adjusted, can injure any other abdominal organ or the spine.

In both belted and unbelted drivers sitting close to the steering wheel, the lower part of the wheel and the hub may strike the epigastrium, resulting in visceral injury. Compression of the pancreas between wheel and vertebral column may cause fracture or contusion of the organ, resulting in enzyme leakage.

Front-seat passengers suffer a similar range of injuries, excluding the effects of impact associated with the steering wheel and pedals.

Restrained rear-seat side passengers are relatively well protected, although impacts with the front seats (usually with the head and knees) may occur in smaller vehicles. However, the centre rear seat passenger usually has only a lap belt for protection, and hyperflexion injury of the spine may occur during impact. Lap belts are commonly not properly adjusted and are worn too high. This not only increases the risk of spinal injury but also the risk of injury to abdominal organs.

Unrestrained rear-seat passengers present a significant threat to the front-seat occupants. The seat backs are relatively soft and will transmit force from a rear-seat passenger's knees to the spine and trunk of the front occupant.

## Oblique frontal impacts

Seat belts are only fully efficient in a square-on frontal impact. Protection may be lost when forces are applied obliquely from the front. For the driver, this effect is most marked if the car is struck on the front nearside, and the opposite for the front-seat passenger. An oblique impact on the driver's side may cause an unrestrained driver's head to be thrown forward against the 'A' pillar (the metal strut running down the side of the windscreen), or against the side window, resulting in severe head injuries.

## Side impacts

Side impacts have the greatest potential of all to produce severe injuries. Such impacts commonly occur when one car emerges from a side road and is hit on the side by another vehicle travelling along the main road; 90° 'broadside' impacts are not uncommon, but most are oblique.

The problem is that the side of the car is relatively weak, with very small distances between the occupant and the outside. There is limited space for energy-absorbing 'crumple' zones. Even if the side of the car could be made rigid and impenetrable, the sideways acceleration of the car and the inertia of the occupant's body during impact would still result in injury. Car sides are not rigid and often some degree of inward intrusion of the damaged bodywork occurs, further reducing or obliterating the clearance between body and car side. At floor level, the car side is quite strong, due to the presence of pressed steel sills that form part of the structure of the car. However, above this the doors are relatively weak, and the impact is taken largely by the vertical 'B' pillar. The low sills of small cars may be overridden by the front of a larger car and thus offer no 'stiffness' as protection against side impact.

Deformation of the side of the car allows force to be transmitted to the occupants, particularly at pelvis level (corresponding to the impacting car's bumper) and to the side of the chest (the grille and bonnet).

The inertia of the head leads to both cervical spine injuries and striking of the head against the side windows or pillars in many side-impact accidents. Strategies adopted by manufacturers to reduce these risks have included the introduction of side air-bags in some luxury models, and stiffening of the side of cars to minimize intrusion.

## Rear impact

Modern vehicles offer quite good protection in rear impacts, even at high speed. Strong seats are essential to prevent spinal injury due to seat collapse, and properly adjusted head restraints help to minimize neck injury.

A stationary car struck from behind will be accelerated forwards. The car's inertia makes this acceleration relatively slow. Some energy is dissipated by the mechanical work involved in deformation of the body work of both cars, and as heat and sound. Parts of the occupant's body strapped to the car (e.g. pelvis and torso) will be accelerated forwards with the car. Free parts (e.g. the head) will retain their inertia. Commonly, people describe their head as being 'thrown backwards' in a rear impact (in reality the head stays where it is as the body moves forward). Hyperextension of the neck and impact of the back of the head with the head restraint (if fitted) occurs. The neck movement may be severe enough to cause excess movement at the cervical intervertebral joints, and avulsion of small pieces of the anterior vertebral bodies. In any case, the cervical ligaments are stretched and post-crash neck symptoms are common.

Head restraints are intended to be energy-absorbing and severe head injuries are uncommon. However, with a heavy occupant the loading on the seat may be severe, resulting in the structure collapsing backwards. In this situation, the occupant is relatively unprotected by the seat belt and may be ejected from the seat into the rear of the car, resulting in injuries to the head and spine.

Where there is no effective head restraint, even low-velocity impacts result in hyperextension injuries to the neck. Following hyperextension, the head often 'flops' forwards again into pronounced flexion—this mechanism being known commonly as 'whiplash'. Additionally, the car may be shunted forwards into the back of a third vehicle, thus creating a secondary deceleration and neck flexion, an event that increases the risk of neck injury.

### Roll-over

As discussed previously, seat belts are only fully effective in frontal impacts. In accidents where the vehicle overturns, the seat belt may not restrain the occupant efficiently. During a roll-over, the occupants are subjected to centrifugal forces that cause contact with the side and roof of the vehicle, and also possibly with other occupants. Each of these contacts may cause injury. In addition, failure of the restraints may result in the occupant being partially or completely ejected from the vehicle. A report from the ambulance crew of abrasions and damage to the car roof should be taken very seriously.

## Gunshot injuries

Gunshot wounds, once a rarity in peacetime, are now much more commonly seen in the Accident and Emergency department as a result of the increased use of weapons in crime.

The weapons used to inflict these injuries vary enormously in design, but all fall within one of three broad categories:

(1)   shotguns—firing many small pellets at subsonic velocity;

(2)   low-velocity weapons, including airguns, some handguns, and smallbore rifles, firing a single bullet at subsonic velocity.

(3)   high-velocity weapons, including fullbore rifles.

Although classification of weapons by velocity may be useful to convey a general impression of wounding potential, many more factors are involved in the physics of wounding. The actual amount of energy transferred to tissue, and the behaviour of the missile after penetration are more important factors which influence wounding potential.

Tissue penetration is largely dependent on the mass (affecting momentum) of a projectile, but some missiles deform, tumble or fragment within tissue, and these behaviour characteristics have a major effect on the type of wound caused.

Energy transfer is dependent on both missile velocity and mass, but also on tissue density. There are many cases on record of perforating chest wounds due to high velocity (high energy) missiles which pass through the body without evidence of major cavitation or tissue damage, mainly due to the low density of the lung and consequently the relatively small deceleration effect on the bullet.

## Bullet injuries

Around the turn of the last century, the series of international conventions outlawed the use of 'inhumane' bullets in warfare, which led to the almost universal manufacture of bullets with full copper jackets to prevent flattening and fragmentation within the body. This concept worked well until the latter half of the 20th century, when designers moved towards faster and lighter bullets with thinner jackets. The immense stresses on these high energy projectiles frequently leads to their complete destruction, with secondary fragments dispersed within tissues, and it is important when planning imaging to recognize that such fragments may be found remote from the predicted track of the bullet.

In an over-simplistic way, many textbooks describe low-velocity missile injury as consisting of a simple track through the tissues with no remote effects, and high velocity missile injury to be characterized by cavitation. There is no doubt that cavitation does occur in some high-energy gunshot injuries, but this does not appear to be due to the effects of either a 'shock wave' or to 'missile tumbling'. It is likely to be due to simple physics—the transfer of energy to tissues by the passing missile causing their lateral displacement.

In the early phase after injury, it is unlikely that any imaging modality will demonstrate the full extent of tissue injury in a high energy missile wound, and certainly not the extent of cavitation. For this reason, surgical exploration remains the investigation of choice in most cases. Pre-operative plain radiography and occasionally CT may be helpful in the detection of foreign bodies and the planning of surgery. Vascular injury may not be obvious even at macroscopic inspection of vessels during surgery, and angiography has an important role when questions arise about occult injury.

## Shotgun Injuries

Injuries due to a shotgun discharge may be devastating at close range, due to the high energy of the rapidly expanding plume of pellets and hot gases. However, the many individual small pellets are slowed down rapidly by air resistance, with only superficial tissue penetration at ranges over 40 m and skin penetration unlikely beyond 200 m.

Since widely spread pellets may penetrate the body at different sites, puncturing body cavities and hollow organs, imaging of all affected sites is mandatory—not to detect pellets alone but also to detect complications.

# CHAPTER 5

# Imaging in the patient with multiple injuries

- Key points: imaging in the patient with multiple injuries
- Making the patient safe: the initial clinical assessment
- Investigation of specific areas of the body

---

## Key points: imaging in the patient with multiple injuries

1. The clinical management of life-threatening injuries takes precedence over radiographic assessment.

2. Only vital radiographs which will influence management are done during the initial assessment.

3. The most influential radiographs to be taken in the resuscitation room are:
   - lateral cervical spine;
   - chest;
   - pelvis.

4. Patients should not be removed from the resuscitation area for further imaging until stabilized.

5. If unstable patients have to be moved (e.g. for CT scanning), adequate resuscitation equipment should go with them, along with personnel trained to use it effectively.

6. Large haemothoraces may be missed on supine chest radiographs.

7. All seven cervical vertebrae must be visualized on the lateral cervical spine X-ray. If this is not possible, cervical immobilization must continue.

8. No single form of imaging gives full information about an abdominal injury.

9. Remember the sandwich rule: for example, if there are injuries to the head and chest, there is also likely to be a neck injury; if there are injuries to the chest and pelvis, there is likely to be an abdominal injury.

# MAKING THE PATIENT SAFE: THE INITIAL CLINICAL ASSESSMENT

Severely injured patients may rapidly develop a variety of life-threatening complications, which require prompt action to save life. For this reason, patients are managed in an area with full resuscitation facilities available until their stability is assured. During this phase, very few radiographs are required. Those that influence management should be done within the resuscitation room, if necessary, using a portable machine, and others deferred until later.

Radiology can be integrated successfully into the initial assessment of the patient with major injuries. This assessment falls into three phases, following the principles of the Advanced Trauma Life Support® course:

1. The primary survey:
   A—Airway, with control of the neck
   B—Breathing mechanisms
   C—Circulation, with control of haemorrhage
   D—Deficit in conscious level.

   Any life-threatening conditions are treated as they are discovered. For instance, if a tension pneumothorax is detected clinically during the assessment of breathing, it must be decompressed without waiting for a chest radiograph.

2. The resuscitation phase: during this phase, particular attention is paid to the management of oxygenation, fluid loss, and haemorrhage control.

3. The secondary survey: a detailed head-to-toe examination of the body is performed. At this stage, radiographs of the cervical spine, chest, and pelvis are performed, and decisions are made about which other radiographs and investigations are needed. If deterioration occurs at any stage, the A-B-Cs are revised. When stability has been achieved, other necessary investigations (e.g. full-spine radiographs, limb radiographs, head CT/ultrasound) may be undertaken.

Ideally, a patient should be able to have all investigations performed without being moved. This is only possible with fixed X-ray equipment above the resuscitation trolley, because of the limitations in quality of portable radiographs.

Remember the sandwich rule: for example, if there are injuries to the head and chest, there is also likely to be a neck injury; if there are injuries to the chest and pelvis, an abdominal injury is also possible.

# INVESTIGATIONS OF SPECIFIC AREAS OF THE BODY

The investigations are discussed in order of importance, taking the three mandatory films first—chest, cervical spine, and pelvis. Other body areas follow in the sequence they are examined during the secondary survey.

## The three key images

### Chest

The chest radiograph is the most essential of all in the patient with major injuries. While the decompression of a tension pneumothorax must always depend on clinical evidence rather than waiting for the chest radiograph, the single anteroposterior (A-P) chest film can offer valuable information about other life-threatening injuries.

The film is examined systematically. Examine the soft tissues outside the bony thoracic cage for evidence of surgical emphysema (air streaks). The usual cause for this is a pneumothorax with rib fractures. Examine the two halves of the bony cage for symmetry, and then examine any obvious derangements in more detail. Working from the top, examine both clavicles and the first and second ribs. Fractures to the first rib are reported to be associated with other serious injuries carrying up to 50 per cent mortality. Work down, examining each rib individually. Remember that the liver is located under ribs 5–10 laterally on the right and the spleen under ribs 9–11 posterolaterally on the left. Evidence of rib fractures in these locations should raise serious suspicion of damage to these organs. Similarly, the kidneys are partially covered by the twelfth ribs posteriorly.

The recognition of the presence or risk of a pneumothorax is of great importance, particularly if the patient will require mechanical ventilation. Pneumothoraces in trauma patients are prone to develop tension and may rapidly become life-threatening. If a pneumothorax is suspected (e.g. by the presence of surgical emphysema), look carefully at the lateral heart border for evidence of air between the heart and lung, and look above the clavicles for loss of the normal lung markings. An expiratory chest radiograph may lower the clavicles enough to allow the edge of the pneumothorax to be seen.

The interpretation of portable supine anteroposterior chest radiographs requires caution. Large amounts of blood may collect behind the lung under gravity in a thin layer which initially has only subtle effects on the radiographic appearances. Again, asymmetry is a clue not to be missed.

A supine chest radiograph in a patient with bilateral chest injuries just before death was misinterpreted as 'normal but under-penetrated'. In fact, at post-mortem over 3.5litres of blood were found distributed between the two sides of the thorax. Even though both sides of the chest were affected, asymmetry in appearances could be seen.

Finally, examine the diaphragmatic domes. Air-filled cavities lying above the shadows of the domes are indicative of diaphragmatic rupture. Free air beneath the diaphragm indicates damage to one of the hollow organs within the abdomen, but this may not be obvious on a supine film.

More subtle changes are discussed in Chapter 12.

## Neck

A lateral radiograph of the neck is the next priority and gives information about both soft tissues and the bony cervical spine. Adequate films, showing down to the C7–T1 junction are not always easy to obtain due to the large bulk of tissues in the shoulders obscuring the view. The reject rate of lateral cervical spine films is double that of films for most other body regions. To maximize the chances of obtaining an adequate film on the first exposure, the patient's arms are routinely pulled down towards the feet to depress the shoulders. This may not be possible if the patient has painful injuries to the upper limbs. A further or alternative measure is to abduct one arm beyond 90° in order to obtain a 'swimmers view' radiograph of the lower cervical area via the axilla. Again, this technique is both painful and potentially hazardous if the patient has shoulder or upper-arm injuries, and certainly if an unstable injury of the cervical spine is present.

The lateral film is examined as follows. The film is quickly scanned for gross abnormalities. The integrity of the line running down the anterior surface of all of the cervical vertebrae is examined, followed by that of the posterior surfaces. A further line marking the posterior margin of the spinal canal is examined, followed by the shape of each of the vertebral bodies and of the spinous processes. The soft-tissue shadows in front of the vertebral bodies are examined and the presence of any gas noted. The lucent space marking the position of the airway is examined for narrowing by soft-tissue encroachment.

The soft tissues in front of the vertebral bodies are usually 5 mm thick or less above the larynx and less than the thickness of a vertebral body below the start of the oesophagus. Widening of the soft tissues may indicate the presence of a fracture haematoma in the locality.

Detailed assessment of any abnormalities found is discussed in Chapters 9 and 11.

## Pelvis

Fractures and disruptions of the pelvis may not be apparent on examination but lead to major haemorrhage, often requiring massive blood replacement. A pelvic radiograph is essential in the diagnosis of unexplained shock and forms part of the minimum image set for all multiple injury patients.

When examining the anteroposterior pelvis film, look for symmetry between the two sides. The pelvis is normally a complete ring—follow the contour of the bowl of the pelvis to look for interruptions in the ring. Any damage to the ring normally occurs in two places, not one (just as a Polo mint always breaks in two places). Thus, a disruption of the symphysis pubis is usually associated with either a fracture through both rami or the ilium on one side or a disruption of one sacroiliac joint.

Examine the pubic rami closely, then the blade of the ilium on both sides, then the acetabular contours for continuity. When a pelvic disruption is suspected, look also for an avulsion of the fifth lumbar vertebral transverse process, which may be pulled off by the tough iliolumbar ligament. The width of the sacroiliac joint is variable, depending on the projection, but should be equal on both sides.

The application of angiography and interventional radiology to the management of major pelvic haemorrhage is discussed in Chapter 7.

# Further imaging

## Skull

Patients with a depressed conscious level due to head trauma rarely benefit from an immediate skull radiograph series. Computed tomography offers more diagnostic information and is the investigation of choice. The only indication for urgent skull radiographs is in those patients who have evidence of penetrating injury to the cranium. Radiographs may then demonstrate free air, foreign bodies, and in-driven bone. Findings on CT scanning in head trauma are discussed in more detail in Chapter 9.

## Facial bones

Major fractures of the facial bones may compromise airway stability, and action will have been taken during the primary survey to correct this. Both distortion of normal anatomy and major haemorrhage present immediate threats to life and these are dealt with before imaging can be considered. On the initial radiographs, facial symmetry is the first important consideration, followed by examination of the film for the presence of fluid in the facial sinuses—a sign that often points to significant bony injury. A systematic check of the contours of the orbits, facial sinuses, zygomata, and maxilla, followed by the mandible, is performed. Finally, the nasal bones are examined in both planes. Radiographs may give an important indication of whether any teeth have been broken or avulsed—in an unconscious patient these potential foreign bodies must be looked for on the chest film.

## Abdomen

Conventional radiography of the abdomen in the injured patient is not normally a priority, and offers little diagnostic information except in the case of gunshot and bomb-blast injuries, where foreign material might be found.

If the patient is unstable, the most appropriate early investigation for suspected intra-abdominal injury is diagnostic peritoneal lavage. This will usually assist the decision on whether the patient will need an immediate laparotomy. However, the investigation offering most diagnostic information is CT scanning, and this is preferable if it is available and if the patient has been stabilized successfully. Ultrasonography and contrast imaging may be helpful in selected cases.

## Limbs

Obvious fractures of the lower-limb long bones are normally dealt with by the application of traction splintage early in the management of the injured patient. Early plain radiographs do not therefore influence management decisions. The exception is a finding of posterior dislocation of the hip, which will be obvious from the pelvic radiograph anyway. Dislocation of the ankle also requires prompt treatment but this is largely a clinical diagnosis.

Clinical evidence of circulatory problems, including loss of foot and ankle pulses, indicates the need for angiography as soon as the patient is stable enough to be moved, after life-threatening injuries have been managed. Some patients may require angiography in the operating theatre while surgical procedures are being undertaken to control haemorrhage and repair injured vessels.

# CHAPTER 6

# The imaging of foreign bodies

.................................................................................................................................................

- Key points: the imaging of foreign bodies
- Sites of foreign bodies
- The techniques available
- Bibliography

**Key points: the imaging of foreign bodies**

1. The range of foreign bodies that may be found lodged in the body is immense. The resulting symptoms and signs will depend on the characteristics of the objects and their location. Imaging is frequently needed for the diagnosis and treatment of these cases.

2. Choosing the most appropriate imaging modality and the right views to order for conventional radiography is important in the diagnosis of retained foreign bodies.

3. For the detection of radiopaque foreign bodies by conventional radiography, the purpose of the investigation must be communicated to the radiographer, as the exposure chosen is often very different from that used for detecting bony injuries.

4. Ultrasonography is useful for the detection of superficially located radiolucent foreign bodies such as wood, and isodense foreign bodies such as aluminium and plastics.

5. CT is useful for detection and location of foreign bodies in areas of complex anatomy such as neck, orbit, and brain.

## SITES OF FOREIGN BODIES

A foreign body in the airway can result in an immediate life-threatening situation, but those in the gastrointestinal tract or soft tissues more often result in delayed morbidity. Although the range of clinical symptoms can be wide and at times confusing, there is nearly always a preceding history of foreign body inhalation, ingestion, or wounding, and a high index of suspicion on the part of the doctor is valuable. In suspicious cases, appropriate and skilful use of the available imaging modalities in any hospital, however rudimentary, can prove beneficial.

## Foreign body (FB) of the eye

Traumatic injuries to the eye resulting from both penetrating and also apparently blunt mechanisms can introduce a foreign body into the globe or orbit. Evidence of ocular penetration or a puncture wound of the globe deserves further evaluation.

Conventional radiography of the orbits, including anteroposterior and lateral views, is usually obtained as the initial investigation after history taking and thorough physical eye examination. In the majority of cases, this would aid in establishing the presence of a foreign body.

In highly suspicious cases, or in the obvious acute injury to the orbit, CT is the method of choice. The value of CT lies in its ability not only to detect the presence of a foreign body but also to locate it precisely and to determine its relation to the surrounding vital structures in the orbit. This obviously has significant importance with regard to the planning of surgical treatment.

Ultrasonography, however, does not play an important role in the evaluation of the acutely injured orbit. The presence of a gas bubble introduced from a puncture wound may occasionally mimic a foreign body, thus leading to confusion in diagnosis.

The possibility of the foreign body being metallic precludes the use of MRI as an imaging modality to evaluate suspected foreign bodies in the eye. However, MRI, with superior soft-tissue discrimination, has a role in the evaluation of blunt orbital trauma if there is no risk of metallic FB.

## Foreign body of the ear and nose

History and physical examination are usually sufficient to establish the diagnosis of retained foreign body in the ear canal or nose. Radiological imaging is therefore generally not required. On the other hand, foreign bodies left in these orifices for a protracted period may lead to infection of the surrounding structures. CT of the ear may be required to assess the temporal bone for such complications.

# Foreign body of the airway

Inhalation or aspiration of a foreign body can have a wide range of presentations, ranging from sudden life-threatening symptoms to none at all. Quite frequently it is the later secondary complications, such as chest infection, which lead the patient to seek medical advice. Fortunately, in the majority of patients there is sufficient time for a proper diagnostic work-up.

The traditional method of making the diagnosis is to obtain a chest radiograph. Even if the foreign body is radiolucent, there are indirect features on the chest radiograph to indicate the presence of a foreign body beyond the carina. These initial changes are secondary to ball-valve effects of the foreign body in the airway, resulting in air trapping. Air enters the lung on inspiration but fails to escape on expiration.

Inspiratory- as well as in the expiratory-phase chest radiographs are taken, and may show little or no change in the volume of the affected lung between phases, whereas the normal side expands on inspiration and reduces in volume on expiration. To demonstrate air trapping in a restless patient, fluoroscopy can be an alternative. However, if the obstruction is complete, the affected lung may show complete collapse within a short period of time after the impaction.

The diagnosis of foreign body aspiration in children usually starts with a high index of suspicion. Such children frequently have unilateral hyperinflation or atelectasis on the chest radiograph. It is important to note that in the first 24 hours the chest radiograph may appear normal. When the foreign body is of vegetable matter a consolidation may be seen instead, because organic matter tends to cause significant local inflammation.

If the foreign body is located in the larynx of a child, a frontal view will prove more useful than a lateral projection of the neck. Overlapping laryngeal structures may obscure small foreign bodies or simulate the appearance of one.

Foreign bodies lodged in the trachea commonly produce symptoms of both upper- and lower-airway obstructions. These are not difficult to diagnose, since a fairly large foreign body is required to cause obstruction of the wider airway, while smaller ones pass on further into the bronchial tree. More often than not they produce discernible opacity, identifiable on the frontal chest radiograph alone.

Overlying anatomical structures, such as the great vessels and thymus, seen on the frontal chest radiograph may obscure the foreign body in the trachea, especially in an underpenetrated film. A lateral radiograph may prove more valuable.

While it is possible to diagnose inhaled foreign bodies with sophisticated imaging techniques, it may be preferable in highly suspicious cases to save time by proceeding to bronchoscopy. The advantage is that bronchoscopy can be both therapeutic as well as diagnostic. When bronchoscopic expertise is not available and plain radiographs are equivocal, computed tomography may locate the foreign body and be of assistance when deciding whether to transfer the patient to a specialist unit.

## Foreign body in the gastrointestinal tract

Ingested foreign bodies that are commonly seen in A&E practice are often found lodged in the pharynx, oesophagus, stomach, small and large intestines, including the rectum. Clinical features are important, including the site of discomfort, presence of a dental plate (which reduces the ability to feel bones in the food bolus), the inability to swallow fluid after the onset of symptoms, and any history of choking. Some impacted foreign bodies are life threatening; for example, button batteries ingested by children and drug packages ingested by smugglers.

### Pharynx and oesophagus

Foreign bodies often lodge in the normal anatomical points of narrowing. Therefore in a child both the airway and gastrointestinal tract must be evaluated. This will include chest and abdominal radiographs.

Fish bones are common sharp objects that may impaled in the wall of the pharynx or cervical oesophagus. A lateral cervical radiograph taken using a soft-tissue technique will demonstrate most radiopaque foreign bodies. On the other hand, demonstration of non-opaque foreign bodies relies on the presence of soft-tissue swelling or gas introduced in the prevertebral soft tissues as indirect signs.

In the oesophagus, the majority of foreign bodies are seen lodged at the thoracic inlet, but may also be found at the level of the aortic arch, the crossing of the left main bronchus, or the gastro-oesophageal junction. A posteroanterior (P-A) chest radiograph may suffice, but if this is non-diagnostic a lateral chest radiograph is also required. Dentures lodged in the lower oesophagus behind the heart may be obscured in the frontal view but more evident on the lateral view.

Children less than 2 years old are generally very inquisitive and are prime candidates for unsuspected oesophageal foreign body. A foreign body lodged in the upper oesophagus may present to the physician with symptoms of upper-airway obstruction, the reason being that the child's trachea is softer than in the adult and more prone to extrinsic compression.

Aluminium foreign bodies (e.g. ring-pull tabs from cans of drink) are extremely difficult to detect on a plain radiograph. Unless either the physician has a high degree of suspicion from the history, or complications such as perforation are already present, the aluminium foreign

plain radiograph, which is readily available in the A&E department, should be obtained, and is the imaging modality most commonly relied upon. Two views are usually obtained perpendicular to each other. An opaque marker made from a paper clip may be placed at the puncture site to add value to the plain radiograph for assessment of the distance and angle of the foreign body from the puncture site. The majority of foreign bodies are radiopaque, showing up as a radiolucent filling defect, or have an air halo that makes detection easier. However, the radiographer must be told the purpose of the examination, since choice of exposure is often very different from that used to detect bony injury.

The demonstration of a foreign body depends largely on its density, size, and orientation. The main limiting factor appears to be the size of the radiopaque foreign body. Fragments as small as 0.5 mm can be detected on standard radiographs when unobscured by underlying bone, but otherwise the foreign body may have to be at least 2 mm in size to be detectable.

It may be almost impossible to identify isodense (similar density to surrounding soft tissue) foreign bodies, such as aluminium and some plastics, on plain radiographs. Other imaging modalities, such as ultrasound or a metal detector, are required.

## Ultrasonography

The increasing availability of this modality in A&E departments makes ultrasonography a useful adjunct to conventional radiography in the detection of radiolucent (wood) or isodense (aluminium) foreign bodies. High-frequency probes of 5 MHz or higher are required to detect a superficially located foreign body. The detection depends on the difference in the acoustic impedance between the foreign body and the surrounding soft tissue. This results in the reflected sound beam from the interface being represented as an echogenic structure, or cast an acoustic shadow.

Metallic and glass foreign bodies are most reflective. Wood fragments are hyperechoic and may produce acoustic shadowing. Unfortunately, wood tends to decompose rapidly and becomes less echogenic with time. Plastics generally are also echogenic and can demonstrate acoustic shadowing.

## Computed tomography

The advantage of multiple planar imaging and the ability not only to discriminate, but also to provide spatial orientation of, the foreign body from the surrounding soft tissue, makes CT the modality of choice, especially in areas of complex anatomy such as the neck, orbit, and brain. This advantage is especially apparent when other imaging modalities fail to detect or locate the foreign body and suspicion remains.

Unfortunately, the cost of CT, coupled with greater radiation dose when compared to conventional radiography, makes it unsuitable as a routine screening examination to detect foreign bodies or as a screening test for objects of unknown composition.

## Magnetic resonance imaging

Although MRI shares many advantages and disadvantages with CT, to date the role of MRI in detection of foreign bodies is unclear. Although no radiation is involved, any likelihood or suspicion of a ferromagnetic foreign body is a contraindication for this examination. However, when there are no contraindications and other modalities have failed to identify the suspected foreign body, magnetic resonance imaging has proven useful.

## Special cases

### Gunshot wounds

Gunshot wounds involving the vital organs commonly result in death, but for those who survive to reach emergency care, imaging plays a central role in detecting the extent of wounding and of complications. Missiles may variously halt intact, exit the body, disintegrate, or hit bone and cause secondary injurious fragments. Determination of the fate of the bullet or fragments is important in the planning of operative débridement of the wounds.

Bullet wounds to the head require preparation of a careful imaging plan. The first priority is, as always, to stabilize the general condition of the patient. If a decision to continue with resuscitation and active management is made, the investigation of first choice is CT to assess the extent of intracranial bleeding which may lead to increased intracranial pressure and circulatory compromise. Plain skull radiograph also has a place in the early management as it avoids the streak artefacts that are created on CT by the bullet. Plain radiographs allow the number and position of fragments to be determined, assisting the neurosurgeon in planning the operative approach.

Another consideration is the possible contamination of gunshot wounds with pieces of cloth, hair, and other materials that may become embedded along the wound track when a bullet passes through the clothing the patient is wearing. Lack of awareness of this possibility may lead to development of infection that cannot be resolved despite aggressive antibiotic treatment.

Intrathoracic and intra-abdominal gunshot wounds can be assessed quickly from a plain radiograph. When the patient's condition permits, CT can be used to determine the exact spatial relationship of the bullet to the surrounding structures, as well as to assess associated injury along the bullet track. Unfortunately, because of the high density of the bullet, some artefacts are unavoidable.

Angiography may be required to identify vascular involvement and therapeutic embolization may be performed to maintain haemostasis.

## Knife wounds

Injuries from knives or any similar offending weapons can be deceptive. Their adverse effects depend primarily on which vital organs are penetrated, but additionally on loss of integrity of fluid and gas barriers.

On inspection the stab wound may appear trivially small on the skin, but will be of indeterminate depth. Adjacent compartments may be involved, depending not only on the depth but also the angle of the stab. A common example would be an upward attack over the liver area where the knife might also pass through the diaphragm into the chest, thus creating a pneumothorax or cardiac wound.

Initially, conventional radiography is used in the assessment of penetrating intrathoracic injuries. An erect chest radiograph offers most information and may be permissible if the patient is conscious and has no apparent mechanism of neck or spine injury. Whereas a haemothorax of 200 ml or less can be missed on an erect radiograph, even larger amounts of blood may collect without any clear change being seen on a supine chest radiograph. A decubitus film with the patient lying on the affected side might help to confirm clinical suspicion if the patient cannot be sat up.

Alternatively, ultrasonography can be performed and the typical anechoic collection characteristic of acute bleed may be seen in the pleural space.

Unfortunately supine chest radiography also makes the detection of a pneumothorax difficult. Pneumothoraces in the supine position tend to accumulate anteriorly and are easily missed, even when fairly large in volume. Careful scrutiny of the supine chest radiograph for subtle signs can help. These include the contours of the mediastinum on the affected side appearing clearer and sharper in outline, and the anterior diaphragm may appear depressed.

Injuries to the heart can be rapidly lethal, usually from blood loss but also when the presence of haemopericardium leads to cardiac tamponade. A quick ultrasound scan in the cephalad direction from the xiphisternum can help to detect the presence of fluid in the pericardium. At the same time ultrasound can be used to place the needle accurately for immediate pericardiocentesis to relieve the tamponade.

In an otherwise stable patient a bedside ultrasound examination can be performed which may detect intrathoracic or intra-abdominal collections from a visceral rupture or bleeding. However, detection of bowel perforation may be difficult.

When clinical examination and imaging results are equivocal or a mismatch exists between symptoms and clinical findings, spiral CT can be performed. In the majority of stable patients who sustain chest or abdominal injuries, CT can help to make management decisions about whether a conservative approach or a laparotomy is necessary.

Even with negative imaging results, it is prudent to observe patients with knife wounds to the chest or abdomen for a period of time. This allows a repeat of the appropriate radiological imaging should symptoms persist or worsen.

# BIBLIOGRAPHY

Ballinger PW. Merrill's Atlas of Radiographic Positions and Radiologic Procedures, 8th edn. Missouri: Mosby, 1995; 1:501–18.

deLacey G, Evans R, Sandin B. Penetrating injuries: how easy is it to see glass (and plastic) on radiographs? Br J Radiol 1985; 58:27–30.

Hollerman JJ, Fackler ML, Coldwell DM, *et al.* Gunshot wounds: 1. Bullets, ballistics and mechanisms of injury. AJR 1990; 155:685.

Hollerman JJ, Fackler ML, Coldwell DM, *et al.* Gunshot wounds : 2. Radiology. AJR 1990; 155:691.

Kuhns DW, Dire DJ. Button battery ingestions. Ann Emerg Med 1989; 18:293–300.

Litovitz T, Schmitz BF. Ingestion of cylindrical and button batteries: an analysis of 2382 cases. Pediatrics 1992; 89(4 Part 2):747–57.

Little CM, Parker MG, Callowich MC, *et al.* The ultrasonic detection of soft tissue foreign bodies. Invest Radiol 1986; 21:275–7.

Selivanov V, Seldon GF, Cello JP, Crass RA. Management of foreign body ingestion. Ann Surg 1984; 199:187–91.

Steinbach BG, Hardt NS, Abbitt PL, *et al.* Breast implants, common complications and concurrent breast disease. Radiographics 1993; 13:95–118.

Steiner RM, Tegtmeyer CJ, Morse D. The radiology of cardiac pacemakers. Radiographics 1986; 6:373–5.

Wechster RJ, Steiner RM, Kinori I. Monitoring the monitors: the radiology of thoracic catheters, wires and tubes. Semin Roentgenol 1988; 23:61–84.

# CHAPTER 7

# Specialist techniques and interventional radiology in trauma

- Key points in interventional radiology
- The techniques available
- Use in specific injuries
- Bibliography

---

## Key points in interventional radiology

1. Diagnostic angiography and interventional techniques are applicable in a wide range of traumatic conditions, but cases require careful selection.

2. Apart from vascular intervention, interventional techniques have been developed for some other injuries, for example in the urinary tract.

3. Appropriate interventional techniques have reduced the need for immediate surgery, and offer definitive treatment in instances when surgical treatment is not practical or possible. They may assist in preparing and planning a subsequent surgical approach.

---

## THE TECHNIQUES AVAILABLE

Both penetrating and blunt trauma may cause injuries to the local vasculature. Signs and symptoms, particularly from soft-tissue injury, may be absent or masked by those of other injuries. To ensure optimal patient outcome in major trauma, it is essential to determine the critical injuries that have the most significant consequences in order to select definitive and reliable diagnostic studies and institute appropriate treatment.

In most cases, treatment involves immediate or early surgery. However, some injuries are amenable to non-surgical treatment and, occasionally, surgery may be contraindicated. In these situations, interventional radiology has a therapeutic role.

Interventional radiology offers both diagnostic and therapeutic management options. Improved techniques, better equipment, and greater safety have contributed to a more successful outcome.

Angiography is initially performed to determine the integrity of vascular anatomy, and also to further delineate the extent of the vascular injury. Subsequently, when the source of bleeding is identified, embolization can be performed either as an exclusive therapy or as an adjunct to surgery. Often it is simpler, cheaper, and more tissue sparing than surgery.

Many post-traumatic and postoperative collections or abscesses are now easily drained percutaneously using interventional radiological techniques. In addition, percutaneous stenting is nowadays commonly performed in the postoperative management of complications of biliary and urinary trauma.

# USE IN SPECIFIC INJURIES

## Vascular injuries

Vascular injuries may be due to compression by a structure or bleeding, spasm, or intimal dissections and tears. These may lead to displacement, occlusion, thrombosis, or haemorrhage.

Victims with complete transection of the aorta are often dead before arrival in the Accident and Emergency department. On the other hand, complete avulsion of an arterial branch may lead to spasm and result in temporary cessation of bleeding. An injured artery can bleed into a cavity, surrounding tissue or, less commonly, into another vessel, resulting in a fistula, the latter often developing days or weeks after the initial traumatic event.

Venous injuries are generally considered secondary in importance to arterial injuries. Often injuries involving the small- and medium-calibre veins are not treated beyond securing haemostasis. However, injuries to major veins, such as the venae cavae or their main tributaries, can be lethal. These injuries are often diagnosed on the operating table rather than in the angiographic suite.

Occasionally, a foreign body may find its way into a major artery, causing occlusion and producing symptoms largely depending on the extent of the narrowing of the lumen.

# Neck

Injuries to the neck are mainly due to penetrating mechanisms, and most will require either angiography or surgical exploration. However, penetrating injuries that do not extend through the platysma often do not require further evaluation.

Zone I injuries (see page 102) require emergency surgery for control of haemorrhage. Currently, there is a tendency for more patients to be evaluated by preoperative angiography to improve the accuracy of diagnosis and for better planning of the surgical approach.

Zone II injuries involving the common carotid arteries and internal jugular veins are easily accessed surgically due to their superficial location. The vertebral arteries, on the other hand, are surrounded by bone and associated soft-tissue structures, which hinder clinical assessment and often limit surgical access. Therefore evaluation of the vertebral arteries by angiography proves to be a better initial strategy than surgical exploration.

Zone III injuries are almost nearly always inaccessible to the surgeon and require angiographic assessment. If necessary, transcatheter embolization can be performed during angiography to control bleeding. This is the method of choice for treating injuries of the vertebral and external carotid arteries.

# Chest

Injuries to the thoracic aorta and other intrathoracic segments of the brachiocephalic arteries must be considered in all cases of significant blunt trauma to the chest.

Mechanisms of injury that are associated with vascular damage include:

(1) rupture at the isthmus of the descending thoracic aorta as a result of a frontal collision at high speed with the patient unrestrained;

(2) partial tear in the lesser curvature of the distal arch above the isthmus may result from a broadside collision;

(3) avulsion of the innominate artery from the aortic arch as a result of direct mechanical injury from a fracture.

Most patients with obvious signs would be operated on immediately on arrival. However, the few that are haemodynamically stable, and patients with equivocal clinical features of great-vessel injuries, will generally benefit from preoperative aortography to identify injuries to the aorta and the main branches.

## Abdomen and retroperitoneum

Organ preservation and control of haemorrhage are the major objectives in the management of intra-abdominal and extraperitoneal haemorrhage. The liver and the spleen are the most frequently injured, most commonly by laceration. These wounds may be superficial and stop bleeding spontaneously. Although deeper and more complicated lacerations are often repaired at emergency surgery, embolization may be performed postoperatively as an adjunct to the initial surgical arterial haemostasis.

Early diagnosis and treatment of avulsion of the renal pedicle by reimplantation or grafting may salvage the injured kidney. Intrarenal arterial haemorrhage causing irreversible segmental renal damage may be treated by superselective embolization.

Traumatic rupture of the renal pelvis or ureter may be managed by non-vascular interventional techniques such as percutaneous nephrostomy and antegrade ureteric stenting, allowing healing to occur without operative intervention.

Lumbar arteries may be torn in either blunt or penetrating trauma. Haemorrhage from these vessels is often difficult to treat surgically, and surgery carries a high risk of iatrogenic nerve root injuries. Diagnosis and treatment may be made easier with the use of angiography, together with embolization techniques.

## Pelvis

Pelvic fractures with disruption of the ring are often associated with massive haemorrhage. This is a major cause of death among victims with major pelvic fractures. It is essential to assess the volume of blood loss, severity and source of haemorrhage, and angiography is often performed to localize the bleeding site and to assess the extent of injury.

Embolization can be used to control the haemorrhage while the patient is still in the angiography suite. This has proved helpful in the control of bleeding, as demonstrated by a significant reduction in the need for blood transfusion after embolization.

With improved techniques in diagnostic angiography and therapeutic embolization, this approach is becoming widely accepted as the procedure of choice to localize bleeding vessels in major pelvic trauma prior to an aggressive surgical approach.

Surgical exploration in the presence of pelvic fractures can produce fatal results, as the exploration of the retroperitoneal space may relieve the tamponade effect on bleeding vessels, leading to further uncontrollable haemorrhage. Furthermore, identifying the bleeding vessels intraoperatively in the presence of extensive haematoma is almost always impossible.

The arteries most vulnerable in pelvic fractures are the superior gluteal, lateral sacral, internal pudendal, and obturator. Arterial injuries are most prevalent in the following pelvic fractures:

(1)   anteroposterior compression types II and III;

(2)   lateral compression type III;

(3)   vertical shear; and

(4)   combined mechanisms.

Injuries of the superior gluteal and lateral sacral arteries are commonly associated with fractures of the ilium and sacrum, or with the separation of the sacroiliac joint. Bleeding from the internal pudendal and obturator arteries are associated with diastasis of the pubic symphysis or fractures of the pubic rami.

Fortunately, bleeding from visceral arteries from blunt trauma is relatively uncommon, but may accompany penetrating injuries.

Complications from embolization are generally rare. Potential risks of impotence and footdrop have been reported.

## Limbs

Vascular injuries of the limbs frequently occur as a result of motor vehicle and industrial accidents. A high clinical suspicion of vascular injury is aided by recognition of the '5 Ps': pain, paralysis, paraesthesia, pallor, and pulselessness.

Some fractures and dislocations are particularly prone to vascular complications. These including those around the knee, affecting the popliteal vessels, and fractures of the supracondylar humerus, injuring the brachial artery. On occasion, vascular damage can occur distant from the immediate vicinity of the skeletal injury, particularly if distortion of the limb occurs as part of the injury mechanism.

## Conclusions

Diagnostic angiography and interventional techniques are appropriate in a wide range of trauma cases. In many situations, appropriate and timely radiological intervention has reduced the need for surgery.

## BIBLIOGRAPHY

Allison DJ, Wallace S, Machan LS. Interventional radiology. In: Grainger RE, Allison DJ, eds. Diagnostic Radiology : an Anglo-American Textbook of Imaging. Edinburgh: Churchill Livingstone, 1992; 2329–90.

Ben Menachem Y. The mechanism of injury. In: Ben Menachem Y, ed. Angiography in Trauma. A Working Atlas. Philadelphia: WB Saunders, 1981; 25–46.

Ben Menachem Y, Handel SF, Ray RD, Childs TL, III. Embolisation procedures in trauma: the pelvis. Semin Interv Radiol 1985; 2:158–81.

Brown JJ, Greene FL, McMillin RD. Vascular injuries associated with pelvic fractures. Am Surgeon 1984; 50:150–4.

Chait P. Future directions in interventional paediatric radiology. Pediatr Clin North Am 1997 Jun; 44(3):763–82.

Dodd GD, Esola CC, Memel DS, *et al.* Sonography: the undiscovered jewel of interventional radiology. Radiographics 1996 Nov; 16(6):1271–88.

Feliciano DV, Herskowitz K, O'Gorman R, *et al.* Management of vascular injuries in the lower extremities. J Trauma 1988; 28(3):319–28.

Fisher RG, Ben Menachem Y. Embolisation procedures in trauma: the abdominal—extraperitoneal. Semin Interv Radiol 1985; 2:148–57.

Gibbon WW. Interventional radiology techniques in musculoskeletal disease. Baillières Clin Rheumatol 1996 Nov; 10(4):711–27.

Kadir S. Diagnostic Angiography. Philadelphia: WB Saunders, 1986; 382.

Kam J, Jackson H, Ben Menachem Y. Vascular injuries in blunt pelvic trauma. Radiol Clin North Am 1981; 19:171–86.

McCorkell SJ, Harley JD, Morishima MS, Cummings DK. Indications for angiography in extremity trauma. AJR 1985; 145:1245–7.

Mallory D, McGee W, Shawker T, *et al.* Ultrasonic guidance improves the success rate of internal jugular vein cannulation. Chest 1990; 98:157–60.

Pachter HL, Spencer FC, Hofstetter SR, *et al.* Experience with selective operative and nonoperative treatment of splenic injuries in 193 patients. Ann Surg 1990; 211(5):583–91.

Sclafani SJA. Angiographic control of intraperitoneal haemorrhage caused by injuries to the liver and spleen. Semin Interv Radiol 1985; 2:139–47.

Sclafani SF, Florence LO, Phillips TF, *et al.* Lumbar arterial injury: radiologic diagnosis and management. Radiology 1987; 165(3):709–14.

Selby JB Jr Interventional radiology of trauma. Radiol Clin North Am 1992 Mar; 30(2):427–39.

Uflacker R, Paolini RM, Lima S. Management of traumatic haematuria by selective renal artery embolisation. J Urol 1984; 132:662–7.

# CHAPTER 8

# Non-accidental injury (child abuse)

- Key points: non-accidental injury
- Clinical aspects
- The use of imaging
- Bibliography

---

### Key points: non-accidental injury (NAI)

1. The diagnosis of NAI requires an exceptionally high index of suspicion, and radiological investigation forms only part of the diagnostic process.

2. Epiphyseal–metaphyseal injuries are the most characteristic finding and metaphyseal fractures of long bones are believed to be almost pathognomonic of NAI, especially in a child who is not yet walking.

3. Often a simple fracture with an inappropriate history or at an unusual site is encountered and may alert the doctor to the possibility of NAI.

4. The detection of multiple bony injuries of different ages is suspicious.

5. Although skeletal surveys may be indicated in the investigation of possible NAI, they should not be ordered routinely in the A&E department.

---

## CLINICAL ASPECTS

Child abuse is a major social issue and, when suspected, it is often necessary to use imaging techniques to establish and document the diagnosis. This is important for both medical and legal reasons, because if left undiagnosed, continued abuse may lead to permanent physical and psychological damage and even death. The psychological sequelae that may occur in the long term may not be apparent to clinicians in the early stages.

By far the most dramatic presentation of child abuse is injury due to physical abuse. Other forms of abuse, namely sexual abuse, emotional abuse, physical neglect, and Münchausen syndrome by proxy are often less dramatic and can be difficult to detect.

In the majority of cases, it is often possible to distinguish non-accidental injuries from accidental ones. This requires a detailed history of the traumatic event and a careful analysis of the radiological findings. Historical clues to abuse include delay in seeking medical help, inconsistent or conflicting histories, and a history that is clearly implausible. A high index of suspicion is required in identifying these cases.

Generally there is no single criterion that can be used in isolation to make a definitive diagnosis of child abuse. However, the presence of predisposing factors, presence of physical indicators, and imaging findings can together help to determine whether a child has been physically abused. Predisposing factors to child abuse include previous history of abuse, siblings on the 'at-risk' register', parents who were themselves abused as children, the birth of an unwanted child, or an unwanted pregnancy.

# THE USE OF IMAGING

## The imaging plan in suspected child abuse

Radiology is important in the diagnosis and management of children suffering from physical abuse, but it seldom contributes much to the assessment of children suffering from the other types of abuse. At examination, all injuries should be documented with a detailed description of each injury, as this information often provides the main evidence. Initial radiography in the A&E department should be confined to those images clinically indicated, but certain X-ray findings are highly suggestive of the diagnosis of NAI and warrant further screening of other body areas.

The indications to request a skeletal survey include:

(1)   when the history or injury patterns strongly suggest physical abuse;

(2)   when a history of repeated skeletal injury is present; and

(3)   children in a critical condition with unusual or suspicious circumstances surrounding the injury episode.

Skeletal survey usually consists of the following: two views of the skull, frontal chest and abdomen views, lateral view of the spine (thoracic and lumbar), pelvis, and frontal views of both upper and lower extremities, including the hands and feet. Films taken should be considered potential legal documents.

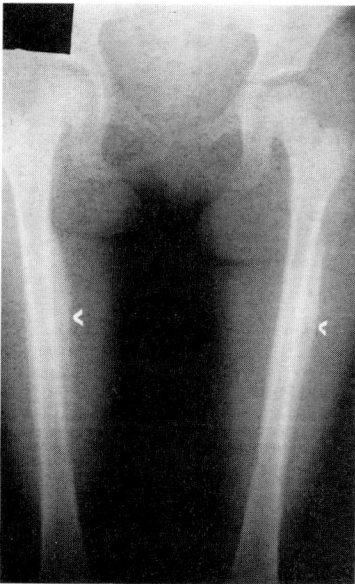

**Fig. 8.1**  Both femora: >, bilateral periosteal reactions along both femoral shafts.

Other radiological studies such as CT, MRI, ultrasonography, and bone scans are sometimes necessary for evaluation of injuries or to confirm suspicious findings on plain radiographs.

When imaging is performed for the above indications, injuries are seen in the musculoskeletal system in 59–80 per cent of cases, central nervous system in 15 per cent, and abdominal cavity in 3 per cent. It is imperative to remember in evaluating skeletal injuries in children less than 5 years old that they differ from adults in several aspects. In young children, the cartilaginous growth plates (epiphyses) are the weakest parts of the skeletal system, whereas the bones are of intermediate strength and the ligaments are the strongest. Therefore, unlike adults, ligamentous tears are less common than disruption and fractures of the epiphyses and underlying bones. The presence of con-siderable amounts of woven bone instead of the adult-type Haversian bone means that bones tend to bend or wrinkle rather than shatter when subjected to stress, and torus or bowing fractures are commonly encountered. In addition, the periosteal membrane is attached loosely to the underlying bone except at the cartilaginous physis and epiph-ysis, and as a result subperiosteal haematoma occurs readily with bony injuries.

Fortunately, in young children, healing and anatomical remodel-ling occur rapidly and often completely. However, in an abused child, proper nutrition and adequate immobilization may be lacking, which may further compromise healing.

## Fracture dating by conventional skeletal radiography

Dating of fractures allows a determination of whether the injury sus-tained is consistent with the history given, and also may ascertain if there have been multiple episodes of skeletal trauma. In general, relatively new fractures can be accurately dated radiographically, but less precision is possible for old injuries.

### 1–3 days

With the initial injury, the fracture line has sharp edges seen on the radiograph similar to those of the edges of a piece of shattered glass. Often there is accompanying soft-tissue swelling which disrupts the normal sharp interface between muscle and subcutaneous fat planes.

### 5–15 days

During this period the fracture line becomes less sharp and more indistinct. This results from bone resorption around the fracture edges. In addition, the presence of slight callus formation often indicates that the fracture is probably 7–14 days old. However, one exception is that rib fractures usually take slightly longer for callus formation to commence—often about 15–20 days.

An unequivocal sign is the formation of calcification in the subperiosteal haemorrhage that appears as periosteal new bone. This can appear as early as 5 days in young infants and in older children should be present by 15 days after the injury.

### 15 days to 6 weeks

It is almost impossible to date the fracture precisely during this period as callus formation becomes more mature and remodelling begins.

### 6 weeks to 8 months

Incorporation of periosteal new bone and remodelling occur. There is often a slight asymmetry of the bony contour that persists for several months and this is often obvious only when comparisons are made with the opposite side. The possibility of a previous fracture can thus be suspected.

In general the following rules are helpful in determining the age of fractures:

(1)   a fracture without periosteal new bone is less than 10 days old;

(2)   a fracture with definite but slight periosteal new bone is more than 10–20 days old;

(3)   a fracture with a large amount of periosteal new bone is more than 2 weeks old.

One area where dating of fractures is particularly difficult is in the skull. This is largely because there is no periosteal new bone formation. However, most skull fractures are visible for a minimum period of 6 weeks but may be invisible or indistinct after 12–16 weeks following the injury. Occasionally, some skull fractures remain visible for months or years.

## Radiological signs of abuse

Certain radiographic findings are highly suggestive of physical abuse. These include:

1.   A single fracture with multiple bruises.

2.   Multiple fractures in different stages of healing.

3.   Multiple metaphyseal or epiphyseal injuries.

4.  Epiphyseal–metaphyseal injuries are reported to be the most characteristic finding in a physically abused child. These often occur in the elbow, presenting as markedly swollen painful joint. Epiphyseal injuries include Salter–Harris type I and II fractures, which in this context are believed to be the result of indirect shearing forces during shaking, twisting, or pulling. Metaphyseal fractures of long bones are common in physically abused children and are believed to be almost pathognomonic of abuse, particularly when they occur in children of the non-ambulatory age group. Unlike the epiphyseal type of injuries, the aetiology of metaphyseal injuries remains obscure. The fractures commonly occur in the knee, ankle, and distal humerus.

5.  Long-bone fractures, particularly the diaphyseal types, are common but can be difficult to distinguish from accidental injuries. In the absence of a history of major trauma, fractures of the femur or humerus are highly suggestive of child abuse. Most of these fractures result from direct blows or torsional forces and present as transverse, spiral, or oblique long-bone fractures.

6.  Fractures of the hands and feet, other than crush injuries of the finger tips, are uncommon in children and if present should raise suspicion. Often a single anteroposterior view each of both hands and feet is included in the routine radiographic skeletal survey.

7.  Rib fractures are rare in children under the age of 5 years unless there is an underlying bone disorder such as metabolic bone disease. In infancy the ribs are very pliable and fractures are often the result of significant force. Fractures occurring from abuse are believed to result from manual compression. Consequently such fractures occur typically in the posterior part of the ribs but may occur laterally or anteriorly along the costochondral junctions. They are often multiple. Rib fractures may be difficult to diagnose radiologically in the acute stages but become more obvious as they begin to heal with callus formation. Clinical features in these cases may prove more valuable. For suspected physical abuse, the routine chest radiograph is a high-yield examination as it allows the ribs, spine, sternum, scapula, acromion, and proximal humeri to be examined in the same film.

8.  Fractures of the sternum, vertebral spinous processes, and scapula are infrequent but when present without a plausible history are highly suggestive of child abuse.

9.  Spinal fractures are relatively rare in abused children. When present, the common types include compression fractures of the

vertebral bodies in the region of the thoracolumbar junction or avulsion fractures of the spinous process. These result from hyperflexion–extension injury involving several consecutive levels. Associated spinal-cord injuries are not common. The lateral view of the spine is best for detecting such abnormalities.

10. Visceral injuries are becoming more commonly recognized in physically abused children. These frequently involve the pancreas and duodenum, liver, spleen, and bladder (the latter being an abdominal organ in early childhood).

11. Skull fractures that cross suture lines, wide (3 mm or more), multiple, complex, and involving both sides of the skull. Head injuries are the principal cause of morbidity and mortality in the abused child, but intracranial injuries may occur either with or without a skull fracture. Presenting features may be varied, including those of raised intracranial pressure or seizures as well as unexplained coma. Further imaging studies may therefore be required to evaluate injuries to the brain accurately in the initial stages.

12. Fractures in unusual locations, such as the occipital bone of the skull.

The important accidental non-intentional injuries of children younger than 5 years include:

1. Skull fractures that are usually narrow and linear, which are not associated with neurological sequelae, these fractures often resulting from a fall onto a concrete or tiled floor and rarely from a carpeted surface.

2. Clavicular fractures are common in children, occurring after a fall onto the arm or the shoulder. These are usually midshaft fractures with variable degrees of displacement.

3. Toddler's fracture is an important accidental injury that is characterized by spiral or oblique hairline fracture of the distal tibia, but which may erroneously raise a suspicion of abuse. Soft-tissue swelling is frequently absent.

4. Greenstick fractures of the radius and ulna.

## Skeletal scintigraphy in child abuse

Bone scanning is generally more sensitive than plain radiographic skeletal survey in establishing physical abuse, due to its high sensitivity for subtle fractures. Typically, scintigraphy becomes abnormal within hours of the fracture. Maximum activity is reached approximately 2 weeks after the injury and gradually reduced over 8 weeks. There are, however, some pitfalls:

1.  Bone scans may fail to detect some fractures, especially those of the skull. This is because most skull fractures are linear rather than depressed. As a result the osteoblastic response is minimal. Skull radiography should be performed instead.

2.  They are of limited value in determining the stages of healing and repair of fractures.

3.  Metaphyseal fractures near the ends of the actively growing bone lie in the regions of maximal normal radionuclide uptake. With poor-quality images, these fractures can easily be missed.

The choice of plain films or skeletal scintigraphy as the primary method of survey for the suspected physically abused child depends largely on the availability of the modality and expertise. Plain radiographs are more widely available and bone scans, although useful, are more often used as an additional study if the plain radiographs show no fractures or show equivocal abnormalities.

Even in cases with almost pathognomonic findings of epiphyseal–metaphyseal fractures, fractures can be found occasionally to be due to rickets, scurvy, multiple congenital contractures, and kinky hair syndrome. It should be borne in mind that underlying disease must be ruled out, either from history, biochemical, or haematological investigations. As with all injuries, a careful history, thorough physical examination, and assessment of the family for any potential risk factors of child abuse should provide the suspicion, if not the diagnosis, of physical child abuse. Imaging forms only part of this total picture.

# BIBLIOGRAPHY

Billmire ME, Meyers PA. Serious head injury in infants: Accident or abuse? Pediatrics 1985; 75:340–2.

Chadwick DL. Child abuse. JAMA 1976; 235:2017–18.

Cumming WA. Neonatal skeletal fractures. Birth trauma or child abuse? J Can Assoc Radiol 1979; 30:30–3.

Harwood Nash DC. Craniocerebral trauma in children. Curr Probl Radiol 1973; 3(3):3–42.

Hobbs CJ, Wynne JM. The sexually abused battered child. Arch Dis Child 1990; 65:423–7.

Kaufman RA, Babcock DS. An approach to imaging the upper abdomen in the injured child. Semin Roentgenol 1984; 19:308–20.

Kleinman PK. Spinal trauma. In: Kleinman PK, ed. Diagnostic imaging of child abuse. Baltimore: William & Wilkins, 1987; 91–102.

Kleinman PK. Diagnostic imaging of child abuse. AJR 1990; 155:703–12.

Kleinman PK, Marks SC, Blackbourne B. The metaphyseal lesion in abused infants: A radiologic–histologic study. AJR 1986; 146:895–905.

Kogutt MS, Swischuk LE, Fagan CJ. Patterns of injury and significance of uncommon fractures in the battered child syndrome. AJR 1974; 121:143–9.

McCort J, Vaudagna J. Visceral injuries in battered child syndrome. Radiology 1969; 92:733–8.

Sty JR, Starshak RJ. The role of bone scintigraphy in the evaluation of the suspected abused child. Radiology 1983; 143:369–75.

Wilkinson RH, Kirkpatric JA Jr. Pediatric skeletal trauma. Curr Probl Diagn Radiol 1976; 6:3–38.

Zimmerman RA, Bilaniuk LT, Bruce D, *et al*. Computed tomography of craniocerebral injury in the abused child. Radiology 1979; 130:687–90.

# PART 3
## *The use of imaging in specific body regions*

# CHAPTER 9

# *The head*

- Key points: the head
- Clinical anatomy
- Clinical assessment
- The techniques available
- Imaging of specific injuries
- Role of cerebral angiography in trauma
- Conclusion
- Bibliography

---

## Key points: the head

1. The presence of a skull fracture is associated with an increased risk of intracranial injury. The purpose of radiographic investigation is to establish whether there is a likelihood of associated brain injury, rather than to demonstrate a fracture.

2. Radiological investigations for the head-injured patient should be performed after the initial clinical assessment has been completed. CT, when available, is the investigation of choice in patients with serious head injuries.

3. Acute intracranial bleeding is often seen as high density (white) on CT, but in patients who are moderately anaemic with a haemoglobin level of 8–10 g/dl, acute haematoma can appear isodense with the rest of the cerebral cortex.

4. Patients with an object impaled in the head (e.g. a knife or nail), should not have the object removed without first identifying the precise location with imaging.

5. MRI should be reserved for instances when CT findings fail to explain the level of neurological deficit. This technique is particularly useful for shearing brain injury.

# CLINICAL ANATOMY

## Skull

The skull is formed by bones of the cranium and the bones of the face and mandible. The cranium is divided anatomically into the vault and skull base: the frontal, parietal, temporal, occipital, sphenoid, and ethmoid bones together form the vault, and the skull base is divided into the anterior, middle, and posterior cranial fossae.

The skull bones are made up of external and internal tables of compact bone, with an intervening diploic space of cancellous bone. The inner table is much thinner and more brittle than the outer table. The neonatal skull has no diploë and has a disproportional large cranium relative to the face.

The cranial cavity contains the brain with its nerves, meninges, ventricles, veins, venous sinuses, and arteries. Differences between these tissues and fluids can be exploited by imaging techniques.

Sutures may form lines, impressions and channels on the vault that are of radiographic significance, and it is necessary to differentiate these normal markings from pathology (Table 9.1, Figs 9.1–9.3).

Vessels are found both closely applied to the skull or within the diploë and appear as lines or channels on radiographs (Table 9.1,

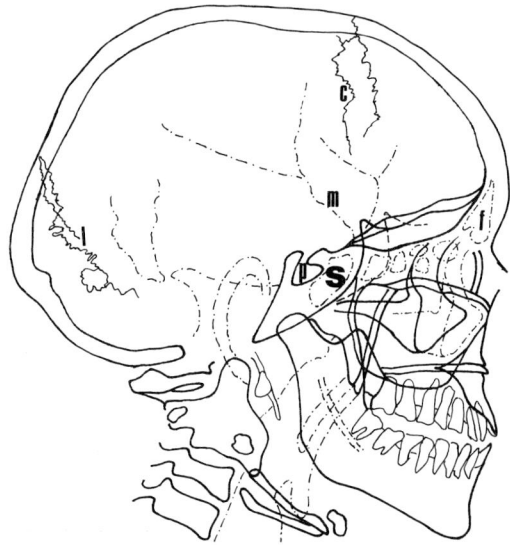

**Fig. 9.1** Skull, lateral view, arterial markings: c, coronal suture; f, frontal sinus; l, lambdoid suture; m, middle meningeal artery impression; p, pituitary fossa; s, sphenoid sinus.

**Table 9.1**   Skull radiograph markings

| Arterial grooves (inner table) | Arterial grooves (outer table) | Venous grooves (diploic veins) | Sutures | Fractures |
|---|---|---|---|---|
| Grooves form on the inner table of the skull | Grooves form on the outer table of the skull | Forms channels in the diploë | Follow a typical anatomical pattern and site | Often involved both inner and outer table of the skull |
| Most prominent grooves are the middle meningeal vessels | Supra-orbital artery—passing superiorly above the orbit | | | May run across anatomical features such as vascular markings and sutures |
| Anterior branch—passing superiorly and posteriorly in front of the pituitary fossa | Middle temporal artery—passing superiorly above the external auditory meatus | | | Paediatric skull—due to the flexibility of the bone only a dent may be visible or may present with an isolated sutural diastasis without a fracture |
| Posterior branch—passing superiorly and posteriorly behind the pituitary fossa | | | | |
| Usually wider than a fracture | | Diploic venous channels are wide | By the age of 3 years the width should be less than 2 mm | |
| Less translucent than a fracture (as only the inner table is affected) | | Less translucent as no inner table is involved | Not as sharply translucent as a fracture line | Straight, translucent line, more translucent when fractures involve both tables |
| Frequently have well-defined white edges | Well-defined white edges | May have a continuous white edge | Fine sclerotic or corticated margins—becoming more apparent with advancing age | Margins are sharply demarcated |
| Tend to branch, becoming narrower peripherally towards the superior aspect of the skull | Appear as straight, narrow grooves | Change very little in calibre throughout their course, wandering course (smooth and undulating, never sharply angled) and irregular confluence | Irregular, serpiginous lines | More straight but can change direction in an acute angle, parallel margins with no tapering |
| Often symmetrical | Often symmetrical | Often symmetrical | Often symmetrical | Asymmetrical |

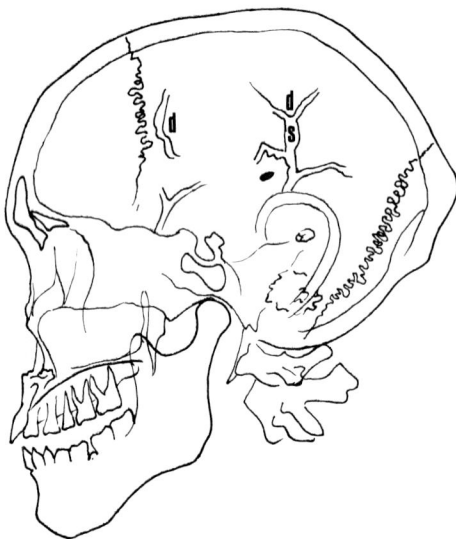

**Fig. 9.2** Skull, lateral view, venous markings: d, diploic veins; s, sinus.

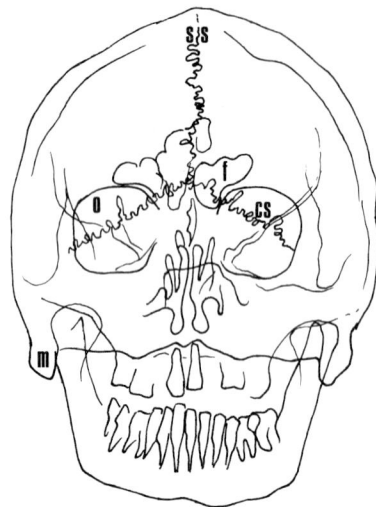

**Fig. 9.3** Skull, frontal view: cs, coronal suture; f, frontal sinus; m, mastoid tip; o, orbit; ss, sagittal suture.

Figs 9.1–9.3). The inner table over these areas is usually thin and may fracture with head trauma, while the outer table remains intact. This may lead to intracranial haemorrhage from adjacent vessels as a consequence of laceration or tear. The superficial temporal artery, which runs in a vertical fashion on the temporal bone may leave an impression that may mimic a linear fracture.

In children vascular markings often only become evident after the age of 2–3 years, and in younger children, the presence of any lucent markings apart from suture lines should lead to the suspicion of a fracture.

Arachnoid (Pacchionian) granulation impressions or granular pits are seen as small, irregular, parasagittal impressions, found adjacent to the superior sagittal sinus.

Several prominent sutures, including the sagittal, coronal, and lambdoid sutures, persist into adult life. At birth these sutures can measure up to 1 cm but by 3 years the normal width will reduce to 2 mm. The two halves of the frontal bone, which normally fuse by the fifth or sixth year of age, may persist instead into adult life. This persistent separation is described as the metopic suture, which should not be mistaken for a fracture. In babies, the anterior fontanelle between the sagittal and frontal sutures is seen on radiographs as a lucent defect and usually closes clinically after 18 months.

Sometimes sutural or Wormian bones are found along the course of a suture (often seen in the lambdoid suture) and should not be mistaken for a comminuted fracture.

Normal calcification within the skull can be visible radiographically. Sites include the pineal gland, habenular calcification, falx cerebri, choroid plexus, petroclinoid ligament, carotid arterial calcification, calcified dura, basal ganglia, and tentorium cerebelli. Externally, the presence of dirt, tightly woven hair, supporting devices such as pillows or folded sheets contaminated with iodine or barium, or film-screen cassette artefacts can simulate intracranial calcification. When in doubt clinical or physical correlation of these findings is essential.

The calcification of the pineal gland appears to have some value in the evaluation of patient with head trauma. In a frontal radiograph of the skull, the calcified pineal gland is seen in 60 per cent of adults, the frequency of visualization increasing with age. If a calcified pineal gland is seen to shift 3 mm or more from the midline in a properly centred A-P radiograph, this suggests the presence of a mass effect from an intracranial lesion. In the clinical setting of head trauma, this would imply significant intracranial haemorrhage. It is essential to ensure that no rotation of the head occurs during positioning for the frontal skull radiograph as this can give the illusion of a pineal gland shift.

## CLINICAL ASSESSMENT

### Indications for investigation

It is essential to determine the mechanism of the injury because more often than not it draws the clinician's attention to the possibility of other associated injuries and possible complications. When the patient is unable to provide an account of how the injury occurred, eyewitness accounts should be sought whenever possible.

Radiological investigations should only be carried out after completing the ABCs of trauma resuscitation as outlined in Chapter 5. Head injuries are known to be particularly associated with neck injury, and stabilization of the neck should be maintained until a cervical injury can be ruled out, either clinically or radiologically.

Abusive or combative behaviour by the patient with head injury may be associated with misuse of drugs or alcohol intoxication, but may also herald a deterioration in the patient's condition due to hypoxia, hypoglycaemia, or raised intracranial pressure.

It is essential that the head-injured patient be monitored carefully for any change in conscious level, as this is the single most important factor in the neurological assessment. The Glasgow Coma Scale (Table 9.2) is a commonly used and internationally accepted means for the evaluation of a patient's consciousness level.

The Glasgow Coma Scale (GCS) is a system of evaluation that is highly reproducible and can be performed by all levels of emergency

**Table 9.2**  Glasgow Coma Scale

|  |  | Score |
|---|---|---|
| Eyes open | Spontaneously | 4 |
|  | To speech | 3 |
|  | To pain | 2 |
|  | Do not open | 1 |
| Best verbal responses | Orientated and converses | 5 |
|  | Disoriented and converses | 4 |
|  | Inappropriate words | 3 |
|  | Incomprehensible sounds | 2 |
|  | None | 1 |
| Best motor response to painful stimulus | Obeys commands | 6 |
|  | Localizes to pain | 5 |
|  | Flexion—withdrawal from painful stimulus | 4 |
|  | Flexes limbs to pain (decorticated rigidity) | 3 |
|  | Extends limbs to pain (decerebrate rigidity) | 2 |
|  | None | 1 |
| Total |  | 15 |

department personnel. An aggregate score of 8 or less is classified as severe head injury, while a score between 9 and 12 is considered moderate and between 13 and 15 as mild head injury. Prognosis for uncomplicated mild to moderate head injury is usually regarded as good. In head-injured patients with a GCS score of 10 or greater, the mortality rate approaches zero if the head alone is involved.

Clinical assessment of the very young head-injured child requires a different set of criteria (Table 9.3), as there is often difficulty in communication and co-operation. However, in children over the age of 5 years the adult Glasgow Coma Scale can be used.

Early and appropriate use of radiographic imaging will lead to a more accurate diagnosis of the head injury and, in most cases, expedite appropriate treatment. In principle, the value of radiographic evaluation of the head-injured patient is to establish whether there is an associated brain injury or a threat of such injury (Table 9.4), ideally accomplished with the least amount of radiation and by the most economic means.

# THE TECHNIQUES AVAILABLE

## Role of conventional skull radiography

Conventional skull radiography has limited usefulness in head-trauma cases. The inability of conventional radiography to provide evidence

**Table 9.3**　Glasgow Paediatric Coma Scale

| | Score | >1 year | <1 year | |
|---|---|---|---|---|
| Eye opening | 4 | Spontaneously | Spontaneously | |
| | 3 | To command | To shout | |
| | 2 | To pain | To pain | |
| | 1 | No response | No response | |
| Best motor response | 5 | Obeys commands | | |
| | 4 | Localizes pain | Localizes pain | |
| | 3 | Flexion to pain | Flexion to pain | |
| | 2 | Extension to pain | Extension to pain | |
| | 1 | No response | No response | |
| | | >5 years | 2–5 years | 0–2 years |
| Best verbal response | 5 | Orientated and converses | Appropriate words and phases | Smiles and cries appropriately |
| | 4 | Disorientated and converses | Inappropriate words | Cries |
| | 3 | Inappropriate words | Cries | Inappropriate crying |
| | 2 | Incomprehensible | Grunting | Grunting |
| | 1 | No response | No response | No response |
| Normal aggregate score | | <6 months | 12 | |
| | | 6–12 months | 12 | |
| | | 1–2 years | 13 | |
| | | 2–5 years | 14 | |
| | | 5 years | 14 | |

**Table 9.4**　Risk of intracranial injury with head trauma

| | |
|---|---|
| Low risk | No symptoms |
| | Headache |
| | Dizziness |
| | Scalp haematoma |
| | Scalp laceration |
| | Scalp contusion or abrasion |
| High risk | Depressed level of consciousness not clearly due to other causes |
| | Focal neurological signs |
| | Decreasing level of consciousness |
| | Palpable depressed fracture |
| | Open wounds with exposed brain or cerebrospinal fluid leak |
| | Post-traumatic seizures |
| | Prolonged unconsciousness following head trauma |
| | Abnormal mental status |
| | Progressive post-traumatic headache |

of intracranial injuries and anatomical detail for subsequent surgical management has made CT the investigation of choice in patients who present with serious head injury. Patients who would benefit from CT evaluation include those with the following clinical features:

- decreased level of consciousness (not definitely due to other causes)

- prolonged unconsciousness following head injury

- decreasing level of consciousness

- abnormal mental status

- focal neurological signs

- palpable depressed fracture

- open wounds with exposed brain

- cerebrospinal fluid leak

- post-traumatic seizures

- progressive post-traumatic headache

- progressive post-traumatic vomiting.

However, as conventional radiography is widely available, is relatively inexpensive to perform, and may be the only imaging technique immediately available, it is more commonly used. Films can be taken quickly in most patients and often do not interrupt monitoring and clinical care. The real importance of identifying a skull fracture is in the associated increased risk of developing an intracranial injury, and conventional radiography remains an important investigation in the less severely head-injured patient.

Some criteria often used for obtaining skull radiographs include:

(1) investigation of penetrating skull injuries for metallic or glass objects of size 0.5 mm or greater (which may cause significant artefact during CT examination, leading to degradation of image quality);

(2) alcohol-intoxicated patients—the skull radiographs may detect fractures early and hence expedite the search for intracranial injury;

(3) children aged less than 2 years;

(4) when other radiological examinations are not possible.

Patients with skull fracture and accompanying altered consciousness have a 25 per cent chance of also having an intracranial haematoma.

# Views to order

The routine views of the skull include the anteroposterior view, lateral view and Towne's view. It is imperative that a patient with a head injury should never be left unattended even for a brief period.

1.   The anteroposterior view demonstrates the orbital margins, the frontal and ethmoid sinuses, sagittal and lambdoid sutures, as well as the diploic veins.

2.   The lateral view (taken either with the right or left side against the imaging plate, depending on the side of injury) shows the frontal and sphenoid sinus, coronal suture, and the middle meningeal artery impression, which divides into an anterior and posterior branch, on the vault.

3.   Often a horizontal cross-table lateral radiograph is performed to demonstrate the presence of a fluid level within the sphenoid sinus or clouding of the mastoid air cells, which in a patient with head injury may indicate a base-of-skull fracture. Usually other special radiographic views are not required if CT is to follow.

4.   The Towne's view (Fig. 9.4), or half-axial view, is contraindicated in patients with suspected cervical injury. This view demonstrates the entire occipital bone, lambdoid sutures, the foramen magnum, and the petrous ridges.

   Skull fractures are more often encountered in adults than in children. On the plain radiographs, common fractures include the linear, depressed, and stellate types. The pattern depends on the age of the patient, severity of blow, the mechanism, and the area of the skull involved.

   Scalp haematomas and lacerations are useful in localizing the point of contact of impact, and also define, in most cases, the potential location of coup and contrecoup injuries.

   The most common fractures seen on the vault are of the linear type. These are usually hairline fractures that generally do not cross suture lines, and most are uncomplicated. However, when fractures involve critical areas such as the middle meningeal artery groove, the deep venous sinuses, or extend into air sinuses, serious immediate or delayed complications may occur. When the linear fracture is not of a hairline type but widely separated, it is more likely to be associated with underlying dural or meningeal tears, subdural haematoma, or cerebral injury.

   Depressed fractures (Figs 9.5, 9.6) usually result from a high-velocity impact injury with an object of small footprint. When see *en face* these fractures show as sclerosis along the edge of the fracture fragments. In the tangential view, the fractured fragment is seen

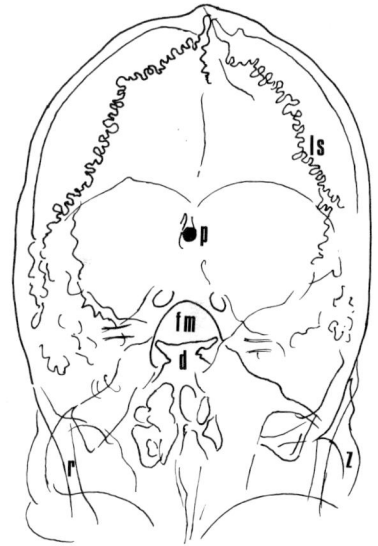

**Fig. 9.4**   Skull, Towne's view: d, dorsum sellae; fm, foramen magnum; ls, lambdoid suture; p, pineal gland calcification; r, ramus of mandible; z, zygomatic arch.

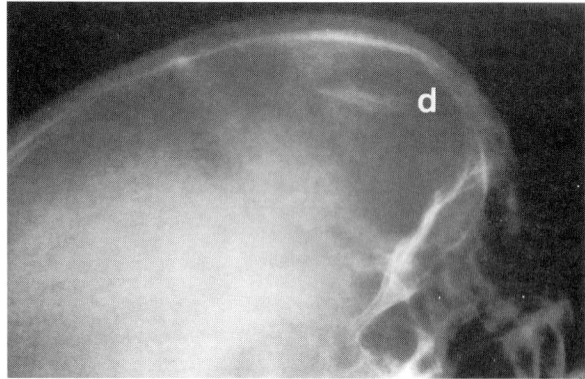

**Fig. 9.5** Skull, lateral view: d, depressed fracture of the frontal bone.

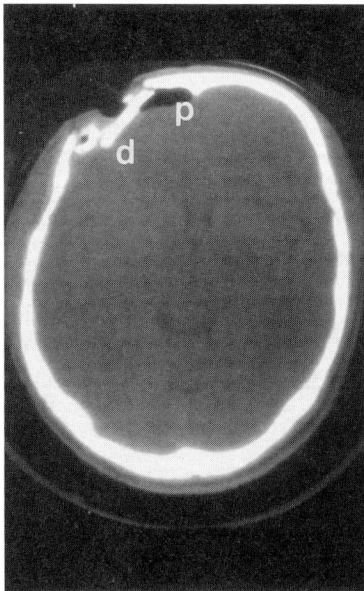

**Fig. 9.6** Skull, CT head (bone window): d, depressed fracture; p, pneumocranium.

depressed and lacks continuity with the rest of the vault cortical bone. A skull fracture depressed 5 mm or more below the inner skull table is more likely to lacerate the dura or cortex. In such cases, CT of the head is mandatory. In children, a localized blow often produces a depression with splintering.

Stellate fractures are so described because fracture lines radiate from the centre of impact. These are usually a form of depressed fracture and tangential views are valuable.

Recognizable clinical signs that help to increase suspicion may accompany fractures of the skull base. Fractures of the petrous temporal bone involving the middle ear and mastoid air cells may produce bruising over the mastoid bone or blood or cerebrospinal fluid leakage in the external meatus. The weakest part of the base of the skull is the middle cranial fossa, because of the presence of numerous foramina, canals, the middle-ear cavities, and the sphenoidal air sinuses in these regions. Basal skull fractures may be complicated by cranial nerve injuries.

Detection of fractures in these areas is often difficult on standard plain radiographs. High-resolution computed tomography is usually required eventually to diagnose and define the actual fracture.

Fractures occurring in the anterior cranial fossa may be clinically evident by the presence of periorbital haematoma, extensive subconjunctival haemorrhage, or nasal cerebrospinal fluid leakage. The majority of injuries result from direct impact to the supraorbital frontal bone or naso-orbital ethmoidal region, or from lateral impact to the anterior face. In such cases, nasogastric tube insertion must be performed with care as, theoretically, the tube may pass directly through the fractured cribriform plate to enter the cranium, with severe consequences.

Penetrating cranial injuries carry an additional risk of depressed bone fragments that may injure the meninges and the brain, leading to significant immediate and delayed sequelae. Penetrating brain injuries will require early surgical exploration to avoid complications such as osteomyelitis, meningitis, cerebral abscess, subdural empyema, and aerocele.

Plaits or beads in the hair or debris contamination can cause artefacts that may mimic penetrating radiopaque missiles or bony fragments. Clinical correlation in most cases readily determines whether the opacities seen on the skull radiograph are artefactual or genuine.

## Role of computed tomography

In the emergency evaluation of the head injured patient CT scanning (Fig. 9.7) is the study of choice. When necessary it can be used to evaluate multiply injured patients who have significant impairment of consciousness and other injuries. The wide use of CT has significantly improved the mortality and morbidity rates for patients with traumatic brain injury, allowing the detection of potentially treatable expanding haematomas or other surgically treatable lesions.

Routine CT scan for head-injured patients usually precludes the use of intravenous contrast. This ensures that fresh haematomas, which appear as hyperdense (white) on computed tomography, are not obscured by the contrast medium. It is necessary to have a protocol that stipulates that images must be taken with a bone window to optimize the detection of fracture, and a soft-tissue window to identify brain injury and, more importantly, the identification of surgically treatable intracranial haematomas. Care should be taken when moving the patient's head, especially when the stability of the cervical spine is unclear. In multiple trauma patients, CT may be used to study more than one region of the body.

In general, a restless patient should rarely be sedated for a CT scan. With sedation, monitoring of the patient's conscious level becomes unreliable and the airway may be compromised if vomiting occurs. Proper general anaesthesia and intubation is a preferable strategy, after checking for obvious causes of restlessness that might be correctable.

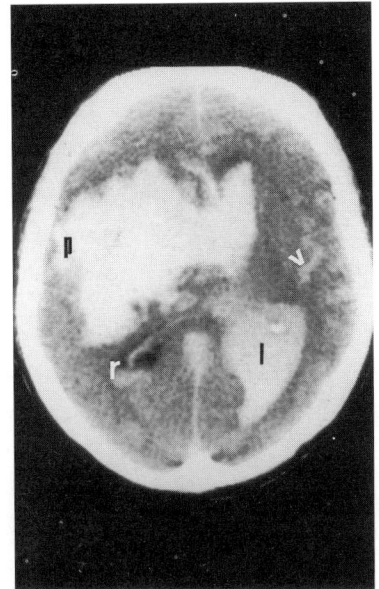

**Fig. 9.7** CT brain, acute massive haemorrhage: Λ, subarachnoid; l, left ventricle, completely filled with fresh blood; p, intraparenchymal; r, right lateral ventricle with fluid level (blood layering in cerebrospinal fluid).

## Role of magnetic resonance imaging

MRI for the head-injured patient should be reserved for those instances when CT findings fail to explain the level of neurological deficit.

Although MRI can provide addition information, in particular the identification of subtle non-haemorrhagic injuries that are often difficult to demonstrate on CT, it often requires a longer scanning time that may delay the required urgent treatment.

**Table 9.5** Magnetic resonance imaging appearance of haemorrhage

| Phase | Composition | $T_1$ | $T_2$ | Comments |
|---|---|---|---|---|
| Hyperacute | Oxyhaemoglobin | High (bright) | High | Hyperacute bleed in <1 hour |
| Acute | Deoxyhaemoglobin Intracellular | Iso | Low (dark) | Deoxygenation Intact hypoxic red blood cells (RBCs) |
|  | Extracellular Methemoglobin | Iso | Iso | After lysis of RBCs Oxidation |
|  | Intracellular | High | Low | After 3—4 days in intact RBCs |
| Subacute | Extracellular | High | High | May be present for months to years |
| Chronic | Hemosiderin | Low | Low | Within macrophages present for years |
|  | Fibrous tissue | Low | Low |  |
|  | Serous fluid | Iso | High |  |
|  | Oedema | Iso | High |  |

MRI, due to its high-contrast resolution, can detect non-haemorrhagic deep cerebral and brainstem contusions or shearing injuries which are often difficult to demonstrate on CT. Also when compared to CT, MRI is superior in detecting haemorrhagic intracranial injuries in the subacute and chronic stages, and small or transversely oriented subdural haemorrhages (Table 9.5).

The disadvantages in the use of MRI in acute head trauma imaging include poor availability, greater cost, incompatibility with ferromagnetic components of life support and monitoring devices, and inability to demonstrate easily pneumocephalus or cranial fractures, including skull-base fractures. Even with a modern MRI scanner, a thorough study of the head-injured patient takes about 15 minutes, which is considerably longer than for a CT scan of the head. In cases of multiple trauma, CT is more efficient when other regions of the body need to be evaluated.

# IMAGING OF SPECIFIC INJURIES

## Cerebral contusion

This occurs when an impact force is transmitted to the brain. When injury to the brain occurs directly beneath the area of impact it is known as coup injury, while that occurring on the side opposite to the cranial impact is known as contracoup injury. A contusion appears on the CT scan as a non-homogeneous area of high and low densities caused by a focal area of mixed haemorrhage, oedema, and necrotic tissue (Fig. 9.8). It is usually accompanied by a change in the patient's neurological status or mental state. CT is usually sufficient to demonstrate this injury although MRI may be able to demonstrate the full extent of the surrounding oedema. Contusions are generally self-limiting but may continue to bleed and form a haematoma, leading to secondary effects.

## Cerebral oedema

Brain swelling resulting from head injury can be focal or global in nature. CT shows an area of low density within the brain substance accompanied by compression or obliteration of the cerebrospinal fluid spaces and sulci. If severe, the swelling may cause a significant mass effect with compression of the lateral ventricles and brain herniation.

## Epidural haematoma (extradural haematoma)

An epidural haematoma develops between the dura and the inner table of the skull. Often it is associated with a skull fracture tearing the middle meningeal artery, but may occur less frequently from tears of the large venous lakes or major dural sinuses. In adults, about 80 per cent of extradural haematomas are associated with a skull fracture seen on the plain radiograph, but the incidence of visible associated fractures is lower in children. As few as 33 per cent of those with epidural haematoma have a history of a classic 'lucid' interval. Mortality rates vary from 7 to 32 per cent in different series.

The haematoma appears on CT as a biconvex or lens-shaped, high-density (white), extra-axial collection that does not cross the sutures (Fig. 9.9). Occasionally, there is a spiral hypodensity within the hyperdense collection. This usually indicates an ongoing bleed in which the fresh bleeding appears as a hypodense area before a blood clot is formed.

As in all cases of expanding haematoma within the limited intracranial space, when the size is large enough, extradural haematoma can produce significant mass effects leading to life-threatening transtentorial herniation. Such haematomas are neurosurgical emergencies and require prompt treatment.

## Subdural haematoma

This is the most common of the extra-axial haematomas seen in the acute trauma setting. Often there are associated cerebral parenchymal injuries giving a prognosis that is usually worse than in those

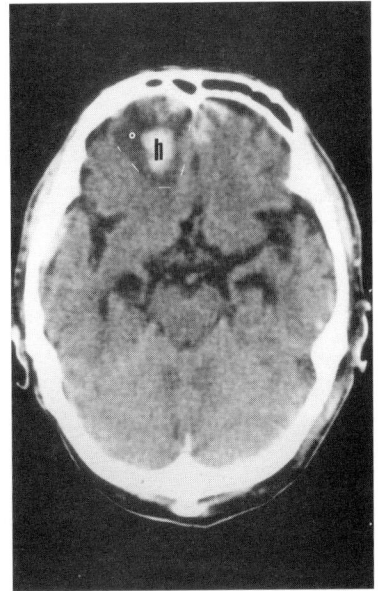

**Fig. 9.8** CT brain, cerebral contusion: h, haematoma; o, surrounding parenchymal oedema.

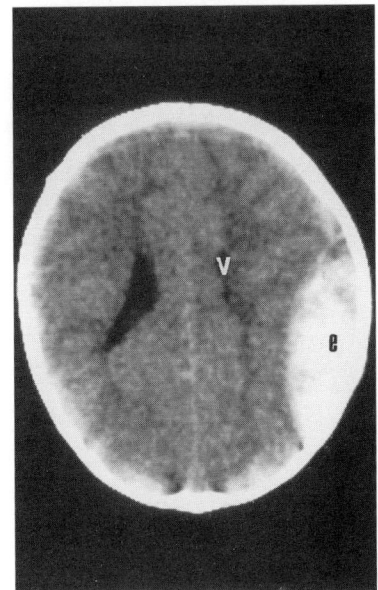

**Fig. 9.9** CT brain, acute extradural haematoma: e, fresh extradural haematoma exhibiting a mass effect with compression of the ipsilateral ventricle (**V**).

suffering from extradural haematoma. The bleeding occurs in the subdural space, which is a potential space lying between the inner layer of dura and the delicate arachnoid membrane.

The injury is usually due to the lag between the movement of the skull and the movement of the brain during acceleration and deceleration. This shearing effect leads to tearing of some of the bridging cortical veins.

Subdural haematoma often appears convex along the inner table of the skull, with a concave inner margin as it conforms to the contours of the brain. Unlike extradural haematoma, subdural haematoma can often occur without a fracture and can cross sutures, but it is limited by the falx and tentorium. It is also separated from the sulci by the intact arachnoid membrane.

The density of the subdural haematoma on CT depends on the time interval after the injury. Acute subdural haematoma less than 24 hours old appears as a high-density area. Subacute haematoma (Fig. 9.10) that presents 2–10 days after the injury appears as a high-density or isodense (density matching the adjacent brain) area. Chronic subdural haematoma, presenting after 10–21 days, appears as an area less dense than adjacent brain.

MRI is generally more sensitive than CT in detecting thin subdural haematomas that occur over the vertex or subtemporal region. It is also more sensitive in detecting blood during the subacute stage, during which, on a $T_1$-weighted sequence, blood will appear bright (white) and the adjacent bone signal will appear black. However, if the patient is anaemic with a haemoglobin level of 8–10 g/dl, even the acute subdural haematoma may appear isointense with cerebral cortex.

In children the presence of subdural haematoma with a poor and inconsistent history should suggest a high possibility of non-accidental injury resulting from violent shaking.

The mass effect of a large subdural haematoma can produce midline shift that is clearly visible on a CT scan. However, when subdural haematoma is present on both sides, midline shift may not occur. Detection of the haematoma is more difficult when the clot is isodense with the adjacent brain and, on occasion, intravenous contrast is given to assist with the identification of the subdural collection. Prompt neurosurgical treatment is required to reduce mortality and improve functional recovery if the haematoma is large enough to produce a mass effect.

Occasionally interhemispheric subdural haematoma may be difficult to differentiate from a diffusely calcified falx. The distinction can be made by the fact that diffuse falx calcification tends to be more irregular and lumpy compared to the smooth outline of the parafalx subdural blood. The other method is to measure the CT density. Fresh blood appears as an area of high density (white) and measures

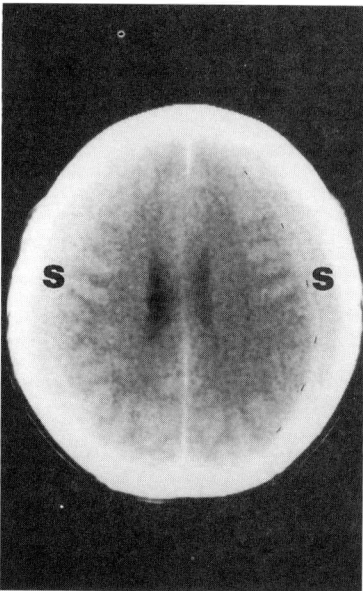

**Fig. 9.10** CT brain, subacute subdural haematoma: s, bilateral haematoma with compression of both cerebral hemispheres.

about 60–90 Hounsfield units (HU) whereas calcification has higher measurements, in the region of hundreds of HU.

It is also common to observe associated injuries, including extradural haematoma, severe contusion, focal or diffuse cerebral oedema, and secondary signs of diffuse axonal shearing injuries. It is important to note that the symptoms of the associated injury may obscure the presence of the subdural haematoma.

## Subarachnoid haemorrhage

Trauma is the most common cause of subarachnoid haemorrhage. Clinically, if the patient is orientated, he will usually complain of headache and symptoms of meningism. In the acute stage, CT appearance is that of an area of increased density extending into the sulci (Fig. 9.11). Cerebral contusion may be seen adjacent to the subarachnoid bleeding.

Occasionally it is difficult to differentiate the aetiology of the subarachnoid haemorrhage. If no obvious evidence of head injury is present, or if the subarachnoid haemorrhage is seen to be isolated in the basilar region, then the possibility of another cause, such as a ruptured berry aneurysm or a bleeding arteriovenous malformation should be considered.

Ten per cent of patients with subarachnoid bleeding will have an apparently normal CT scan. In cases where there is still a high clinical suspicion for subarachnoid haemorrhage, an MRI scan or a bedside lumbar puncture can be performed, although the latter should be performed with extreme care.

Eventually, collections of blood break down and the products appear progressively less dense on the CT scan, until eventually they are absorbed.

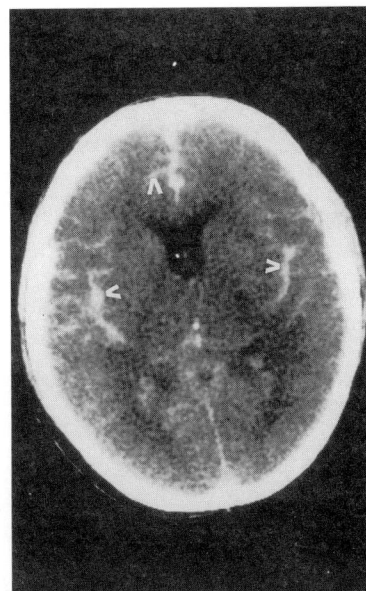

**Fig. 9.11** CT brain, acute subarachnoid haemorrhage: Λ, area of increased density (white) extending into the sulci.

## Diffuse axonal injuries

Shearing within the brain substance resulting from acceleration or deceleration causes these injuries. Disruption of the axons occurs in the corpus callosum, internal capsule, brainstem, basal ganglia, and subcortical white matter. Occasionally, the injured areas may be identified by small petechial haemorrhages.

Clinically, patients usually present with severe neurological deficit and are often found to be unconscious soon after the injury. The comatose state can last for days to weeks, and the overall mortality is about 33 per cent.

CT is not sensitive enough in most cases to detect axonal injuries, except when multiple punctate haemorrhages are also present. These are found in the grey–white matter junction, along the corpus callosum, in the basal ganglia, and in the rostral brainstem

## Brain herniation

Diffuse or focal increased intracranial pressure as a result of haemorrhage or brain oedema can cause herniation of the brain at several locations. Transtentorial and uncal herniations are of major clinical importance. Types that are rarely possible to diagnose clinically include cingulate or subfalcial herniation, which occurs underneath the falx cerebri.

Uncal (medial portion of the temporal lobe) herniation is often heralded by the following clinical sequence: ipsilateral paralysis of the oculomotor nerve, leading to ptosis, mydriasis, and opthalmoplegia; altered consciousness; ipsilateral or bilateral long-tract signs with eventual decerebrate posturing; and ultimately death due to brainstem involvement.

Transtentorial or central herniation refers to downward herniation of both hemispheres and basal nuclei through the tentorium. This often results from an expanding space-occupying lesion, such as haematoma, in the vertex or at the frontal or occipital lobes. The patient may present with altered consciousness, followed by coma and Cheyne–Stokes respiration. As the herniation worsens, both corticospinal tracts may be involved, leading to bilateral muscle weakness which will eventually progress to decorticate or decerebrate posturing.

Both CT and MRI are sensitive and specific enough to demonstrate these brain herniations. However, the easier accessibility of computed tomography make this the imaging modality of choice.

The earliest CT sign of downward (transtentorial) herniation is blunting of the ipsilateral suprasellar cistern, whereas lateral (subfalcine) herniation shows slight arching of the falx and compression of the ipsilateral lateral ventricle.

## Paediatric head injury

The child's skull is more pliable than that of adults and may be depressed sufficiently to cause brain injury without fracturing the skull. The identification of linear, non-displaced skull fractures by conventional radiography has greater significance in children, since intracranial haematomas, tentorial and dural tears, and shearing injuries are more often encountered in young children than in adults. Children with a history of significant head injury, even without evidence of skull fracture, should be admitted for observation. In addition, the potential difficulty in obtaining a reliable history should lower the threshold for ordering skull radiographs in children.

In children aged less than 2 years, clinical hypovolaemia may occur from extracranial bleeding associated with a linear skull fracture. Rapid identification of all injuries is vital, since it is known that young children can make a remarkably good recovery from severe neurological injuries when optimum care and treatment are given and secondary insults are prevented.

Sutural diastasis occurs more frequently in the young infant and child with a closed head injury. This can occur with or without associated fracture of the skull. Diastatic fractures may be associated with haemorrhagic infarcts and leptomeningeal cysts.

## Delayed intracranial haemorrhage

A policy of very early CT scanning after head injury may lead to some haematomas being missed. These can occur as extra-axial or intra-axial haematoma. Most are diagnosed within 48 hours after the injury but may be delayed by up to 2 weeks. Their development is often heralded by a change in the patient's neurological status, and CT is again the ideal imaging modality for detecting such delayed haematomas.

## Post-traumatic cerebral infarction

Infarcts may occur in and around the intracerebral haematoma or as a result of direct compression from an extra-axial haematoma on the cerebral cortex or subcortical region. Unexpected change in the patient's neurological status should prompt repeat CT scanning.

## Post-traumatic cerebral atrophy

This can occur as a focal or diffuse cerebral atrophy. Atrophic changes can be evident on CT as early as 3 weeks after the injury but more commonly these become more obvious after 6 weeks.

## Post-traumatic intracranial infection

Infections are more commonly encountered with open fractures of the skull. Extra-axial empyema, cerebral abscess, or cerebritis can have similar CT features to haematomas that occur in trauma and in patients who have had recent neurosurgical intervention. Their radiological features persist or worsen with subsequent follow-up CT, unlike haematomas which resolve with time.

Epidural empyema is uncommon but, if present, is often seen adjacent to open skull fractures communicating with adjacent sinuses. These empyema collections appear as low-density areas on CT but generally have greater density than cerebrospinal fluid.

Subdural empyema, on the other hand, may have a density equal to or only slightly greater than cerebrospinal fluid. They appear crescentic or lentiform in shape and may be bilateral. CT with intravenous contrast may be helpful in determining the medial border and assist in making the correct diagnosis.

Cerebral abscesses appear as low-attenuation masses on CT, with surrounding oedema. With intravenous contrast the wall of the abscess may enhanced.

## Post-traumatic cerebral tension aerocele

This, fortunately rare, complication may occur after an open skull fracture, especially one involving the frontal sinus, which allows a one-way communication. The air accumulates under tension by a mechanism similar to a tension pneumothorax. Most cases of pneumocephalus are not under tension and resolve spontaneously several days after the injury.

CT is more sensitive in detecting pneumocephalus and can visualize as little as 0.5 ml of gas, whereas skull radiograph can at best detect a minimum of 2 ml. Quantification on serial CT may be necessary if collections are large and when associated with basilar skull fractures.

## Post-concussional syndromes

These occur fairly frequently after head injury and often cause a great deal of anxiety, especially in those who have sustained minor contusional head injuries. The patient commonly presents with headache, dizziness, lack of concentration, depression, and lethargy. Since all of these symptoms can also occur with other head-injury complications, post-concussional syndrome is often diagnosed by exclusion, and CT scanning may be an appropriate interim investigation to detect any treatable cause.

# ROLE OF CEREBRAL ANGIOGRAPHY IN TRAUMA

Vascular complications after head trauma include occlusion, intimal injury, embolism, pseudoaneurysms, and arteriovenous fistulae. If any of these are suspected, cerebral arteriography is performed to detect abnormalities of the cerebral arteries, but it is not without risk.

Cerebral angiography may be necessary when the patient's neurological deficit is not readily explained by the initial CT evaluation. It will help to exclude both intra- and extracranial arterial injuries, and is especially useful when MRI evaluation is not available or is contraindicated.

In patients with an impalement injury of the head, an angiogram is performed after a CT scan to guide the removal of the blade or object by the neurosurgeon.

Cerebral vascular injuries that are not surgically treatable, such as anatomically inaccessible pseudoaneurysms or arteriovenous fistulas, may require interventional angiographic treatment, such as embolization.

## CONCLUSION

In head-trauma patients, there is little correlation between cranial bony injury and the underlying brain damage, and the latter is more likely to be correlated with clinical findings such as coma and neurological deficit. Therefore, clinical examination has a higher value than emergency skull radiography in the head-injured patient. However, there are a few exceptions in which skull radiography is the best investigation, for example to detect metallic foreign bodies, and when a patient's condition or location precludes other examination techniques.

The mainstay of the evaluation of head injury is CT. MRI is also technically an excellent diagnostic modality, in particular in detecting post-traumatic intracranial pathology. However, its inability to demonstrate skull fractures well, and longer scanning time, limits its use in the acute situation.

## BIBLIOGRAPHY

Ballinger PW. Merrill's Atlas of Radiographic Positions and Radiologic Procedures, 8th edn. Missouri: Mosby, 1995; 2:215–69.

Eelkema EA, Heckt ST, Horton JA. Head trauma. In: Latchaw RE, ed. MR and CT Imaging of the Head, Neck and Spine, 2nd edn. St Louis: Mosby Year Book, 1991; 203–65.

Ellis H. Clinical Anatomy, 8th edn. Oxford: Blackwell Scientific Publications, 1992; 341–8.

Frazee JG. Head trauma. Emerg Clin North Am 1986; 4:859–74.

Kleinman PK. Diagnostic imaging in infant abuse. AJR 1990; 155:703–12.

Lee SH, Rao KCRQ, eds. Cranial Computed Tomography and MRI, 2nd edn. New York: McGraw Hill, 1987.

McCort J. Caring for the major trauma victim: the role of radiology. Radiology 1987; 163:1–9.

Masters SJ, McClean PM, Acrarese JS. Skull x-ray examinations after head trauma. Recommendations by a multidisciplinary panel and validation study. N Engl J Med 1987; 316:84–91.

Orrison WW. Introduction to neuroimaging. Boston: Little Brown, 1989; 61.

Smirniotopolis JG *et al*. In: Stuart E, Mirvis, Jeremy WR Young, eds. Imaging in Trauma and Critical Care. Baltimore: Williams & Wilkins, 1992; 23–92.

Snow RB, Zimmerman RD, Gandy SE, Deck MDF. Comparison of magnetic resonance imaging and computed tomography in the evaluation of head injury. Neurosurgery 1986; 18:45–52.

Voris HC. Craniocerebral trauma. In: Baker, Baker LH, eds. Clinical Neurology. New York: Harper & Row, 1982; 1–12.

Zimmerman RD, Danzigan A. Extracerebral trauma. Radiol Clin North Am 1982; 20:105–21.

# CHAPTER 10

# The face

........................................................................................................................................................................................

- Key points: the face

- Clinical assessment

- The techniques available

- Imaging of specific injuries

- Bibliography

---

## Key points: the face

1.  In the initial evaluation of facial trauma, conventional radiography is the modality of choice, providing a comprehensive survey and usually yielding sufficient information for diagnostic purposes with relatively economy.

2.  Multiple views are necessary for evaluating facial injuries in order to reduce difficulty in interpretation due to overlapping structures. These basic views consist of the Waters, Caldwell, and lateral projections.

3.  For adequate evaluation of some regions of the face, it is important to request the right additional views, such as the submentovertex (for the skull base), Towne's, and coned down lateral view.

4.  CT is needed for the diagnosis of some facial injuries, especially when the plain radiographs are non-specific and yet clinical suspicion remains, and for the planning of surgical treatment. Three-dimensional CT is especially useful for planning reconstructive procedures.

5.  MRI is of limited usefulness due to its limited availability and many contraindications. However, with its excellent soft-tissue discrimination, it has a role in the evaluation of blunt orbital trauma.

# CLINICAL ASSESSMENT

Facial injuries are commonly associated with a history of assault or a motor vehicle accident, but may also be caused by accidents in the workplace and in sports. Penetrating injuries are less common but may occur from assault with knives and firearms.

Since the face contains the portals to the patient's airway, severe facial trauma may result in respiratory compromise. Clinical assessment takes priority over imaging techniques, and normally these would only be employed after the secondary survey.

Clinical examination includes inspection for lacerations, depressions, or swellings, and palpation for bony crepitus and deformity. Eye movements are tested in the conscious patient, and in all patients, the maxilla and mandible are tested for stability. Any damage to, or absence of, teeth is noted.

# THE TECHNIQUES AVAILABLE

## Conventional radiography

Information regarding the mechanism of injury from the patient or eyewitness can, on many occasions, direct the examining physician to the specific problem and any possible associated injuries. In addition, it can assist the physician in deciding the types of films to request and the urgency of the request.

Patients who are restless due to alcohol intoxication or head injuries may present difficulty in obtaining good-quality, well-positioned radiographs. Radiographs that are to be of optimal value should have little or no rotation (determined by ensuring that on the radiograph the nasal septum and mandible symphysis are on a fairly straight line, or by tracing the outline of the orbits which should be of the same size and shape). It is better not to waste time and resources if the chance of obtaining adequate films is small.

The adequate plain radiograph can provide a comprehensive survey of the face quickly in the A&E department and is relatively inexpensive. It is usually sufficient for diagnostic purposes and often provides the basic information required for the decision about the need for other imaging modalities.

The routine radiographic series for the evaluation of suspected facial injury consists of multiple views. This is to reduce difficulties in visualization due to overlapping densities on the radiographs. The series consists of Waters, Caldwell, and lateral projections. Additional views are often necessary, including the submentovertex view, Towne's view, and coned down views for nasal bones.

Ideally, the radiographs should be obtained in the erect position to better demonstrate air–fluid levels within the paranasal sinuses. In cases of trauma, this appearance usually indicates haemorrhage from a fracture. Fortunately, the standard views can be obtained fairly easily and are just as informative with the patient in the supine position.

## Waters view

This projection is the single most valuable view and is ideal for evaluation of the midface. It projects the maxillary sinuses above the petrous ridges. It allows adequate visualization of the frontal sinuses, orbital rim and floor, maxillary bone and sinus, and zygoma including the zygomaticotemporal arch.

Although ideally this projection is obtained in the posteroanterior position to minimize radiation to the lens of the eyes, the reverse or anteroposterior Waters view can be obtained when there is a possibility of a cervical spine injury, and in such cases the radiograph can be obtained with the patient in the supine position.

## Caldwell view

In this view the orbital floor projects just above the petrous ridges. It is useful for the evaluation of the frontal and ethmoid sinuses, orbit rim including orbital roof, and the mandible.

## Lateral view

When the erect position is not possible, a horizontal cross-table lateral view should be obtained. This allows visualization of an air–fluid level in the sphenoid sinus which may lead to suspicion of a base-of-skull fracture. This view demonstrates the sphenoid sinus, posterior frontal and maxillary sinus walls, and the pterygoids well. The anterior and posterior walls of the frontal sinus, floor of the anterior cranial fossa, and retropharyngeal soft tissues can also be assessed. Occasionally, concomitant fractures of the upper cervical spine and cranial vault can also be seen.

## Additional views

### *Submentovertex (base) view*
This view is performed with the patient's head hyperextended upon the neck and should not be requested when cervical spine injuries are suspected. When positioned properly, the mandibular symphysis is superimposed on the frontal sinus. This view is obtained primarily when a zygomatic arch fracture is suspected. It is necessary to underexpose this view to visualize the zygomatic arch satisfactorily, and other structures then become difficult to evaluate.

*Towne's view*
This view allows satisfactory evaluation of the mandibular condyles and subcondylar region. In addition it provides information about the zygomatic arches.

*Underpenetrated coned down lateral view of the nasal bones*
The routine lateral view of the face is overpenetrated and is not adequate to evaluate the nasal bones, so a limited further view is needed to examine the nose properly.

*Posteroanterior view of the mandible and bilateral oblique views*
These are performed to evaluate the rami, angle, and body of the mandible.

# Computed tomography

CT is useful both in diagnosis of injuries and in the planning of surgical treatment. In patients with complex facial fractures, CT is able to delineate the presence of fracture and the location of all the fragments. In addition, its ability to discriminate various type of soft tissue further enhances its usefulness.

In circumstances where the plain radiographs appear relatively normal but clinical findings raise suspicion of an underlying fracture, CT is recommended.

In general, both the axial and coronal scans are performed for facial trauma. In cases where cervical spine injury is suspected, coronal images can be obtained from computer reformation from the axial scans, although inevitably some loss of image quality occurs.

Three-dimensional (3D) CT can be reconstructed from the standard axial scans. However, in most cases, 3D CT does not provide additional diagnostic information but can assist in surgical treatment planning, especially for reconstructive procedures.

3D CT is sensitive to slice thickness and there may be a jagged artefact on the reconstructed images when the initial slices obtained are too thick. It is equally important to remember that dental fillings and occasionally endotracheal tubes may cause major artefact, with resultant degradation of the images.

# Other imaging techniques

Ultrasonography has little or no role in the evaluation of acute facial trauma. MRI, because of its limited availability, long acquisition time, and contraindication in patients with metallic foreign body, is of only limited usefulness.

# IMAGING OF SPECIFIC INJURIES

## Nasal bone fractures

The nose, because of its prominent location, is the most frequently fractured structure of the face. The thin, paired nasal bones are attached superiorly to the frontal bone and laterally to the maxillary bones. In adults, the majority of nasal fractures are due to a lateral blow rather than a direct frontal blow.

Often such injuries result in a transverse fracture of the ipsilateral nasal bone and are so obvious clinically that radiographic evaluation for diagnosis is often unnecessary. Clinical examination is more reliable than the radiograph when evaluating the degree of depression of the distal fragment. An exception, perhaps, is when the clinical examination is hindered by the presence of significant soft-tissue swelling.

Radiographic evaluation includes an underpenetrated, coned down lateral view of the nose, which best demonstrates the common transverse isolated fracture of the nasal tip. Occasionally the paired nasomaxillary sutures, or the groove containing the nasociliary nerve which is normally seen on the nasal bone, may be mistaken for the less common longitudinal fractures. However, these normal anatomical markings can usually be differentiated from fractures by their more irregular and less lucent appearance in comparison to a fracture line.

Nasal septal fractures are best demonstrated on Waters view, which allows identification of any displacement or angulation of the septum. The presence of soft-tissue swelling of the nasal septum demonstrated on this view usually represents haematoma. Occasionally, septal injury may lead to complete nasal airway obstruction, especially when there is significant displacement and swelling.

When the injury mechanism is more severe, it is advisable to assess the adjacent bony structures (which include the maxilla, ethmoid and frontal sinus) for fractures. It is also not uncommon for patients to present with associated neurological symptoms such as headache, which may indicate cerebral injury from the same mechanism.

## Frontal sinus fractures

These are frequently the result of a direct blow to the forehead. Frontal sinus fractures may present as a component of a comminuted frontal bone fracture or complicated facial smash injury.

Frontal sinus fractures are often readily visible on the plain frontal radiographs of the face, appearing as lucent lines. When opacification of the frontal sinuses is present, this usually indicates bleeding within the sinus.

Fracture of the posterior wall of the sinus is identified on a lateral radiograph of the face. In such cases, intracranial communication must be considered, as this can have severe consequences if ignored. The presence of pneumocephalus or cerebrospinal fluid rhinorrhea should direct the clinician's attention to the presence of a fracture of the posterior wall of the sinus. CT is frequently required to evaluate not only the sinus but also to identify any intracranial bony fragments and the possibility of cerebral contusion.

# Orbital fractures

Traumatic injuries to the orbits are frequently associated with other facial fractures. In part, this is due to the fact that the orbital walls and rims receive contributions from various facial bones (the orbital contents are protected by seven bones that form the orbital cavity). It is important to note that the thinnest part of the orbit is the floor, which is formed from the roof of the maxillary sinus.

Isolated fractures of the orbit include those involving only the orbital rim or the orbital walls.

## Orbital rim fractures

Isolated orbital rim fractures commonly result from a direct blow to the orbital bony margin but may occur as part of the tripod fracture complex. The site most frequently involved is the inferolateral margin.

Fractures of the superior, lateral, and inferior rim are best visualized with the Waters view whereas the medial and superior rim are seen better with the Caldwell view.

## Orbital wall fracture

Although orbital wall fractures may occur anywhere in the orbit, by far the most common site is the posterior aspect of the orbital floor, or the lamina papyracea of the ethmoid bone (Fig. 10.1).

Blow-out fractures are caused by forces that raise the intra-orbital pressure or push directly on the eyeball itself. Orbital floor blow-out fractures are associated with injury to the medial orbital wall in 20–40 per cent of patients. Isolated blow-out fractures of the orbital roof are rare but are more commonly part of complex craniofacial injuries associated with fracture of the orbital apex. Frontal lobe contusion is almost inevitable in these cases.

### Fracture of the orbital floor
Bruising of the eyelid, subconjunctival haemorrhage, enophthalmos, periorbital oedema, and facial anaesthesia may be found as suspicious

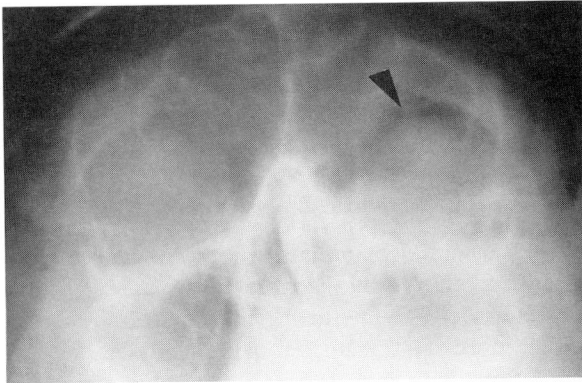

**Fig. 10.1**   Face, Waters view: ◄, left orbital emphysema from fracture of the lamina papyracea.

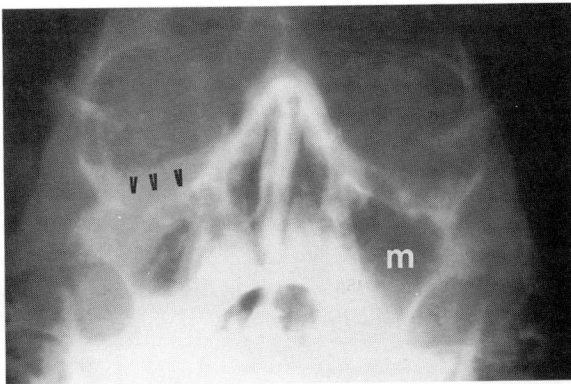

**Fig. 10.2**   Face, Waters view, right orbital floor fracture: v, discontinuity of the orbital floor (maxillary sinus roof); compare to the left maxillary sinus (m).

clinical signs with orbital floor fractures. Diplopia on upward gaze may result from true muscle entrapment but more commonly results from oedema and haemorrhage.

Waters view is recommended to demonstrate the depressed bony fragment of the orbital floor (Fig. 10.2). Opacification of the ipsilateral maxillary sinus usually results from a haematoma. On occasion, it may be possible to see soft-tissue prolapse through the orbital floor, more commonly involving orbital fat than the inferior rectus muscle.

The fracture line is often difficult to identify, but the presence of orbital emphysema almost invariably points to a fracture of the medial orbital wall, and opacification of the ipsilateral ethmoidal sinus is frequently also present.

### Lateral orbital wall fracture

These fractures are difficult to evaluate with plain radiographs and usually require CT for better delineation. However, these are typically associated with ipsilateral zygomatic fractures.

## Further evaluation of orbital fractures

Plain radiographs should be obtained initially because they are relatively inexpensive, offer useful diagnosis information, and they can be performed in the A&E department without excessive patient movement. They are more of a screening tool for orbital fractures, and often more a sophisticated imaging technique is required to obtain a full diagnostic picture.

CT is the method of choice in evaluating all traumatic orbital injuries, especially when patients are at risk for associated intracranial injury, in complex orbital fractures, and for suspected foreign body of the orbit. The advantages of CT include multiplanar axial and coronal images (Fig. 10.3) with the ability to perform three-dimensional reconstruction images, and delineation of fractures difficult to demonstrate by conventional radiography, such as medial orbital wall fractures. The ability to discriminate between various soft tissues, as in the case of soft-tissue prolapse in orbital floor fractures, is an important advantage.

MRI has a role in the evaluation of blunt orbital trauma because of its excellent soft-tissue discrimination, but its limited availability make this a less frequently used imaging modality. The actual or suspected presence of a metallic foreign body in the orbit contraindicates its use.

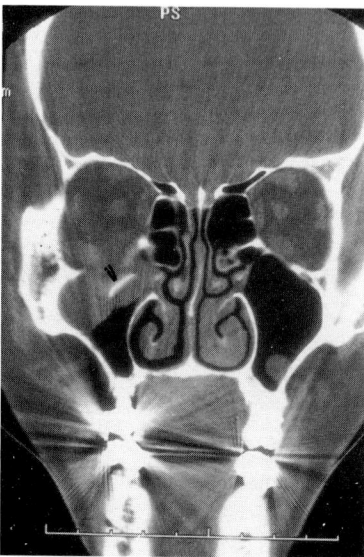

**Fig. 10.3** Face, CT orbits (coronal view): right orbital floor fracture with (**V**) bony fragment in the maxillary sinus.

## Fracture of the zygoma

The cheek prominence is formed by the zygomatic bone, which has a vulnerable position in the facial skeleton. As for other parts of the face, assaults and motor vehicle accidents are the most common causes of zygomatic injuries.

The zygoma articulates with four bones of face, including the maxilla along the inferior orbital margin, sphenoid, the frontal bone at the zygomaticofacial suture, and the temporal bone through the zygomatic arch.

Two commonly encountered injuries of the zygoma are arch fractures and tripod fractures. Fracture fragments are usually displaced inferiorly and posteriorly. Routine plain facial radiograph series are often adequate to identify these fractures.

### Isolated zygomatic arch fracture

A significant localized blow to the side of the face can lead to a depressed fracture of the zygomatic arch. On examination, there is usually accompanying asymmetry of the face, with flattening of the injured side, haematoma, and local tenderness. A palpable depression in the zygomatic arch can be felt when the overlying haematoma is not too large and the patient can tolerate examination.

The routine facial series (in particular the Waters view) can identify disruption of the zygomatic arch. If no contraindications exist, an underpenetrated submentovertex (base) view allows better characterization of the fracture. In this view quantitative estimation of the displacement of the fracture fragments is possible.

Occasionally, bone fragments may be displaced deeply into the temporal fossa and impinge on the coronoid process of the mandible. This presents clinically with difficulty in closing of the mouth and in chewing.

### Tripod fracture

Isolated fracture of the body of the zygoma is rare. Instead, multiple fractures and dislocations usually occur around the sutures.

The fracture involves separation of the body of the zygoma from its frontal, temporal, and maxillary attachments. The following features may be present:

(1) fracture of the frontal process of the zygoma or separation of the frontozygomatic suture;

(2) a fracture of the zygomatic arch; and

(3) a fracture of the maxillary process of the zygoma (including the inferior orbital rim, orbital floor, and the anterior and lateral maxillary sinus wall).

In some cases, the presence of a significantly displaced tripod fracture may lead to diplopia or ophthalmoplegia. Loss of sensation below the orbit may occur if the infraorbital nerve is damaged by a fracture involving its foramen.

The routine facial series is normally sufficient to identify a tripod fracture. The Caldwell or anteroposterior projection is valuable in estimating the separation of the zygomaticofrontal suture. Waters and underpenetrated submentovertex (base) views allow not only the evaluation of the zygomatic arch fracture, but also the orbital rim, orbital floor, and lateral maxillary wall. In addition, the lateral view will also demonstrate any depression, rotation, and displacement of the malar eminence.

CT for the further assessment of tripod complex injuries prior to surgical treatment is advisable.

## Maxillary fractures

The paired maxillary bones form the middle third of the face, also containing the maxillary sinus and upper teeth. Two main types of maxillary fractures are seen—isolated and Le Fort fractures.

### Isolated maxillary fractures

This type of fracture is uncommon and constitutes less than 5 per cent of all midface fractures. The anterolateral wall of the maxillary sinus is most commonly involved and the injury often results from a direct blow to the area.

The Waters view may demonstrate opacification of the maxillary sinus, which in the context of trauma should suggest that a fracture has occurred. The fracture line itself may be difficult to detect but would normally be seen as an abnormal linear density produced by the edge of a displaced fracture fragment.

The Waters view is also ideal for demonstrating dento-alveolar fractures, confirming a clinical suspicion formed on the basis of loosening of two or more adjacent teeth. Attention should be given to the mandible during clinical examination, as there is an associated high incidence of mandibular fracture.

### Le Fort fractures

Although the Le Fort's classification of maxillary fractures is concise and identifies lines of weakness in the face, injuries commonly occur in combination and are typically unstable. According to the classification there are three types of Le Fort fractures (Fig. 10.4).

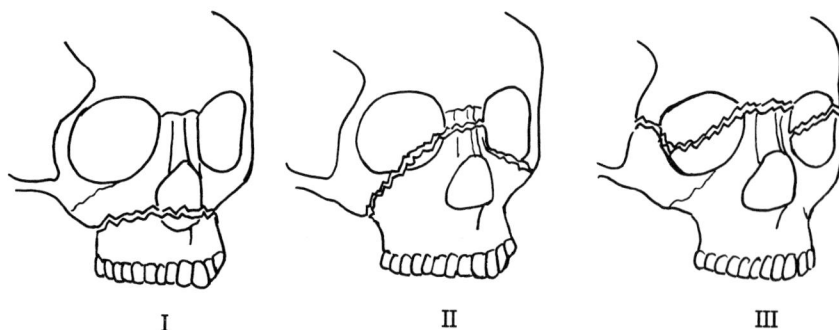

**Fig. 10.4** Face, Le Fort fractures, types I, II, and III.

### Le Fort I fracture

This fracture occurs when a blow strikes the anterior face just below the nose. Clinically, by holding the upper teeth between the thumb and fingers, the teeth are felt to move from side to side.

In Le Fort I fractures the alveolar ridge is separated from the maxilla but there is no involvement of the nasal or the orbital areas. The fracture line includes the alveolar ridge, lateral aperture of the nose, and the inferior wall of the maxillary sinus.

On occasion, even Le Fort I fractures can lead to airway compromise. This occurs when laceration of the palatine arteries results in haemorrhage extending around the inferior constrictor muscles.

### Le Fort II fracture

This fracture occurs when a central force, with or without a downward component, is applied to the face. It is also commonly known as a pyramid fracture due to the separation of a pyramid-shaped loose fragment of the midportion of the face. Clinically the nose tends to move with the teeth. The fracture line includes the arch through the posterior alveolar ridge, medial orbital rim, and across the nasal bone.

### Le Fort III fracture

This is the most complex and severe of all the Le Fort fractures with separation of the entire face from the base of skull. This type of fracture is also known as craniofacial dissociation. Clinically, not only the nose and teeth but also the frontonasal and lateral frontozygomatic areas of the face move together. The fracture line includes a horizontal course through the nasofrontal suture, maxillary frontal suture, orbital walls, and zygomatic arch.

Severe complex facial fractures with severe comminution can occur that do not seem to fit into the classification of any of the Le Fort types of fracture. These have been described very appropriately as facial smash fractures. In these patients it is essential to ensure patency of airway and stability prior to various radiographic examinations, since the investigations needed may be extensive.

The routine facial series, in particular the Waters, Caldwell, lateral, and submentovertex views, would in most cases adequately demonstrate the three types of Le Fort fractures and the main features of the facial smash fractures. However, CT has become essential in the management of patients with complex facial injuries, since good detail of soft tissues and haematomas may be demonstrated. The ability to reconstruct images in various anatomical planes and in three dimensions means that CT has become valuable in the preoperative planning for reconstructive surgery in complex facial fractures.

# Mandible fracture

The mandible is the largest and the strongest of the facial bones, and is second only to the nasal bone in terms of frequency of fractures.

The shape of the mandible resembles a horseshoe or a partial ring, but in reality it behaves like a complete bony ring and fractures often occur in more than one location simultaneously (Table 10.1). For descriptive purposes the mandible is divided into six segments, consisting of the condyle, coronoid process, ramus, angle, body, and the symphysis.

Some fractures are identifiable by the type of injury mechanism. A fall of sufficient force on the chin commonly presents with fracture of the condyles and symphysis. On the other hand, injuries from assault commonly result in fractures of the body and the angle of the mandible.

When the mandible is fractured in children, the injury frequently occurs at the condyles and symphysis. Significant late complications such as occlusal and cosmetic deformities can occur with fracture of the condyles, resulting from growth arrest, avascular necrosis, or bony ankylosis of the temporomandibular joint.

Clinically, most patients with mandibular fractures have an obvious deformity of the jaw. Bruising, external or internal mouth laceration, malocclusion, and pain may accompany this. Fracture of the condyle may preserve normal dental occlusion, but palpation of the mandible externally and from inside the mouth can often detect tenderness, step off, or haematoma from the fracture.

Mandible fractures can be identified easily with plain radiographs that include the posteroanterior and lateral views.

Occasionally, oblique views are obtained as they demonstrate the infracondylar region, coronoid process, rami, and angle of the mandible better. The Towne's view is another projection that may be used to view the condyles, and when there is a need to determine whether there is any displacement of the condyle, the submentovertex view can be employed.

**Table 10.1**  Frequency of fractures of the mandible

| Location of fracture | Frequency of involvement (%) |
| --- | --- |
| Fracture occurring in more than one location | ≈50 |
| Mandibular body and angle | 50–70 |
| Central bony symphysis | 10–20 |
| Ramus | 3–9 |
| Coronoid process | 1–2 |

Any fracture that extends to the teeth must be considered to be an open fracture, especially because of the high prevalence of periodontal disease in most populations.

The directions of mandibular angle fractures are important. When the fracture is orientated posterosuperior to anteroinferior, the opposing fragments are impacted and stabilized by the muscles, but when the fracture occurs in the opposite direction the fragments become separated.

A single panoramic view of the mandible (an orthopantomogram or OPG) can provide additional information but has been replaced by CT wherever this is available. For an OPG, the patient needs to sit erect and has to remain motionless for a relatively long period of about 30 seconds. In many seriously injured patients, this may not be possible.

The use of CT for fracture of the mandible is not routinely indicated but instead it is usually performed as part of a study to assess other facial injuries. An exception is when evaluating the condylar heads for displaced or chip fractures that can be difficult to assess on plain radiographs. In additional, CT allows coronal and sagittal reconstructions, which provide valuable spatial orientation of the fracture and fragments.

Although an uncommon complication, multiple fractures of the mandible can lead to airway obstruction which can be life threatening. This occurs when a 'flail' mandible is present, allowing posterior migration of the tongue and airway blockage, particularly in supine patients who have impaired consciousness. Conscious patients with such injuries often prefer to sit up with the mandible dependent, and become agitated if they are made to lie down on admission to the A&E department.

# BIBLIOGRAPHY

Ballinger PW. Merrill's Atlas of Radiographic Positions and Radiologic Procedures, 8th edn. Missouri: Mosby 1995; 2:299–370.

Cobb SR, Yeakly JW, Lee KF, *et al*. Computed tomographic evaluation of ocular trauma. Comput Radiol 1985; 9(1):1–10.

DeLaPaz R, Brant-Zawadzki M, Rowe Lo. CT of maxillofacial injury. In: Federle MP *et al*., eds. Computed Tomography in the Evaluation of Trauma, 2nd edn. Baltimore: Williams & Wilkins, 1986; 64–107.

Foster CA, Sherman JE. Surgery of Facial Bone Fractures. New York: Churchill Livingstone, 1987; 13–253.

Fuji N, Yamashiro M. Classification of malar complex fractures using computed tomography. J Oral Maxillofac Surg 1983; 41:562–7.

Latchaw RE, ed. MR and CT Imaging of the Head, Neck and Spine, 2nd edn. St Louis: Mosby Year Book, 1991.

Meschan IA. An Atlas of Anatomy Basic to Radiology. Philadelphia: WB Saunders, 1975.

Novelline RA. 3-D imaging of facial trauma. Paper presented at the Second Annual American Society of Emergency Radiology Meeting, 8 April 1991, Clearwater, FLA.

# The neck

---

### Key points: the neck

1. Conventional radiography is the most readily available and cost-effective modality in the initial evaluation of the cervical spine. Portable equipment can be used in the resuscitation area, allowing ongoing monitoring of patients while basic radiographs are being taken.

2. Computed tomography has a cross-sectional imaging capability and images can be reconstructed as sagittal and coronal views. This aids in the diagnosis of neck injuries, assessment of potential instability, and in preoperative planning. However, it is unsuitable for the haemodynamically unstable patient as it usually has to be performed outside of the controlled environment of the A&E department.

3. Magnetic resonance imaging is able to evaluate the soft-tissue components of the neck and spine, but the bony component is poorly demonstrated.

4. Cervical-spine injuries can be safely ruled out clinically when certain criteria are fulfilled, avoiding the need for imaging.

5. Adequate visualization of the cervical spine means that C1 to the C7–T1 junction must be seen on a lateral radiograph and C3 to T1 on the anteroposterior view. Assessment should include the bones and the disc spaces between them, their alignment, and the soft-tissue characteristics.

*(Continued)*

6.  Injuries involving the C1 and C2 are sometimes difficult to assess and indirect radiological clues that indicate these injuries should be sought.

7.  Cervical-spine injuries are less common in children and there are significant anatomical differences between children and adults.

8.  Soft-tissue techniques should be employed if there is any suspicion of airway injury.

9.  The chest may be injured simultaneously in soft-tissue injuries of the neck, and a chest radiograph is essential.

10. Computed tomography is valuable in evaluation of blunt trauma to the airway, being able to define the type and degree of soft-tissue and bony injuries.

11. Angiography is considered the standard approach for the evaluation of zone I and III injuries.

# CLINICAL ANATOMY

The neck is bounded superiorly by the body and the angles of the mandible and inferiorly by the clavicles. It is commonly divided into three zones (Table 11.1) and can be further divided into two triangles by the sternocleidomastoid muscles—the anterior and posterior triangles (Table 11.2).

Muscles of the neck are compartmentalized into seven fascial planes. Trauma to the soft tissue is often apparent by haemorrhage or swelling and, if severe, is often accompanied by pain and restricted movement.

**Table 11.1**  Zones of the neck

| Zone | Anatomical regions | Remarks |
| --- | --- | --- |
| Zone I | Below the cricoid cartilage | Injuries in this zone carry the highest mortality because of major thoracic structure involvement |
| Zone II | Between the cricoid cartilage and the mandible | Most common zone injured in penetrating injuries. Haemorrhages are easily controlled by direct pressure and are accessible to surgical exploration |
| Zone III | Above the angle of the mandible | Injuries to this zone involve major vessels, the aerodigestive tract, and salivary glands |

**Table 11.2**  The anterior and posterior triangles of the neck

| Division | Structures | | |
|---|---|---|---|
| | Vascular | Neural elements | Glands |
| Anterior triangle | Facial artery<br>Internal carotid artery<br>External carotid artery<br>Internal jugular vein | Facial nerve<br>  (cervical portion)<br>Glossopharyngeal<br>  nerve | Submandibular<br>  gland<br>Thyroid gland |
| | Remarks: major vessels<br>  frequently injured by<br>  both blunt and<br>  penetrating trauma lie in<br>  the anterior triangle | Vagus nerve | |
| Posterior triangle | External jugular vein<br>Subclavian artery | Dorsal scapular nerve<br>Thoracic nerves<br>Spinal accessory nerve<br>Brachial plexus | |

## The cervical spine

A typical vertebra is made up of a body, the transverse processes on each side, the pedicles, the laminae, the superior and inferior articular processes, the spinous process, and the pars interarticulares which are situated between the two articular processes. The seven cervical vertebrae are linked by both ligaments and discs. The first cervical vertebra (atlas) and the second (axis) differ in shape and size from the remaining vertebrae.

The vertebral body only has a definitive radiological appearance after puberty in the cervical region, the anterior height being lower than the posterior height, and this should not be interpreted as compression.

The dens, or odontoid peg, of the axis (C2) and its stabilizing horizontal ligament allows rotation between the atlas (C1) and axis. Except for the atlas, the transverse processes of all the cervical vertebrae have a foramen that allows the vertebral arteries of each side to pass upwards to the skull base.

Topographically, the C1 vertebra is usually located immediately behind the angle of the mandible, the hyoid bone is anterior to the level of C3, the thyroid cartilage is located anterior to C4, and the cricoid cartilage anterior to the C6 vertebra.

The cervical segment of the spinal cord is cushioned from trauma by spinal fluid and epidural fat. The vertebral canal tends to be triangular in shape and is relatively larger in this region compared to the thoracic region. The eight paired cervical spinal roots exit through the intervertebral foramina.

# THE TECHNIQUES AVAILABLE FOR IMAGING CERVICAL-SPINE TRAUMA

Once the routine cross-table lateral cervical-spine film has been performed, the choice of imaging techniques to evaluate the patient suspected of having a cervical-spine injury is dependent on the patient's condition. A clear understanding of the role and capabilities of the available imaging modalities is vital.

## Conventional radiography

This is perhaps the most cost-effective, and in some instances the only possible, means of initial radiological evaluation of patients with acute spine injury. This modality has the advantage of being readily accessible, quickly available and, most importantly, portable, therefore allowing it to be performed in the resuscitation area of the A&E department. It also allows the optimum overview evaluation of the whole cervical spine and is frequently specific and definitive.

## Conventional tomography

This modality has largely been superseded by computed tomography, but it still has a place in situations where CT is not readily available. Patients need to be repositioned in order to obtain tomograms in anteroposterior and lateral projections, which is not always possible, and the amount of radiation is greater than that used in computed tomography.

## Computed tomography (CT)

CT is a high-yield imaging modality for the neck due to its cross-sectional imaging capability. It is commonly used to further evaluate the area of suspected injuries detected on plain radiographs. It is able to evaluate both the bony and soft-tissue components, and to assess the spinal canal for any impingement by bony fragments while the patient's spine remains immobilized. Sagittal and coronal image reconstructions aid in diagnosis, assessment of potential instability, and preoperative planning.

One of the main disadvantages is that CT often has to be performed outside the controlled environment of the A&E department and requires the co-operation of the patient to remain still in order to prevent motion artefacts. Horizontal fractures and displacement in the sagittal plane may not be completely evaluated, especially with conventional CT.

## Magnetic resonance imaging (MRI)

This modality has many advantages, including the exquisite ability to evaluate non-invasively the soft-tissue components of neck and spine, which include the intervertebral disc spaces, sites of ligamentous injury, haematoma, and spinal-cord injury. However, it is poor in the evaluation of bony components when compared to conventional tomography or CT.

Indications for MRI would therefore include clinical evidence of spinal-cord injury without plain radiographic evidence of bony abnormality, and assessment of soft-tissue and ligamentous injury which CT cannot differentiate from the normal. There is difficulty in imaging patients who are critically ill and on life support, where the equipment may not be compatible with MRI. The long scanning time required and limited availability in many hospitals are additional factors that limit its use.

## The use of conventional radiography in major trauma

In patients who have sustained major trauma, the immediate priority is to identify and treat immediate life-threatening conditions and to immobilize the cervical spine simultaneously. Cervical-spine injury is always assumed to be present in major trauma patients, and the entire spinal column is immobilized at least until fractures can be reliably ruled out. If immobilization has been initiated in the prehospital setting, it is important to re-check that the immobilization is effective. Immobilization of the cervical spine is by means of a backboard and a combination of hard collar, sand bags, and tape or head wedges. During the secondary survey of the multiply injured patient, the cross-table lateral cervical film should be the first radiograph to be performed. However, several studies have shown that the lateral view is inadequate as the sole view in screening for cervical-spine injury, and therefore the anteroposterior and open-mouth odontoid views should be obtained before abandoning immobilization—together these three views improve the detection rate of abnormalities to approximately 95 per cent.

In some clinical situations, cervical-spine injury can be excluded clinically and therefore a request for radiographs may not necessary. For clinical exclusion of cervical-spine injury the following criteria should be fulfilled:

(1) A patient whose mental status is unclouded and not affected by head injury, drug or alcohol intoxication, excessive anxiety, psychiatric, or medical conditions.

(2) The patient is able to communicate well with the doctor and fully comprehend what is being said to him or her.

(3)   There is no complaint of neck pain of any kind at any time after the trauma.

(4)   There is no other major injury that causes more pain, enough to distract the patient's attention, to obscure cervical pain.

(5)   There is no tenderness to palpation on clinical examination.

(6)   There is no neurological disorder of the trunk or extremities.

The following conditions should increase suspicion of the presence of cervical-spine injuries:

(1)   The presence of depressed level of consciousness in a major trauma patient.

(2)   The mechanism of injury involved high-energy transfer to the head or neck regions.

(3)   The presence of neck pain, numbness, paraesthesia, or weakness of the extremities.

(4)   The presence of head, neck, and facial injuries.

(5)   In the paediatric patient who has suffered multisystem injury, where pain from other injuries may mask neck pain and tenderness.

(6)   The presence of flaccid extremities in a conscious paediatric patient should be assumed to be due to spinal-cord injury.

In all patients with suspected cervical-spine injury, adequate visualization of all seven cervical vertebrae on the cross-table lateral view is essential. Some manoeuvres can be performed to improve visualization on the lateral view. These include applying traction on the patient's arms downwards towards the feet to depress the shoulders, or the use of the swimmer's view (Chapter 5). One other view that can assist in the visualization of the lower cervical spine is the supine oblique view, and this may be helpful in selected patients for the evaluation of unilateral locked facets and posterior laminar fractures or subluxations. The advantage is that the neck need not be moved.

Special radiographic studies may be required after the initial evaluation with the standard views. If there is no contraindication to moving the neck, flexion and extension views may be requested for the assessment of ligamentous integrity. In acute injuries of the cervical spine these studies should only be obtained after neurological and radiological consultation and should be performed by experienced staff.

## Interpretation of conventional radiographs

The cervical-spine radiograph should be assessed and interpreted in a systematic order, and proper radiographic interpretation is dependent upon both the quality and adequacy of the films. One important principle is that all seven cervical vertebrae must be fully visualized, including the C7–T1 junction.

Routine examination of the cervical spine includes a lateral view, an anteroposterior view and, in the conscious patient, an open-mouth view to demonstrate the odontoid process. The most common sites for cervical injuries are the C1, C2, and C5–C7 regions. Extra attention should be paid to these areas. Evidence of disruption of the anterior or posterior spinal ligaments or interspinous ligaments, with or without loss of alignment, indicate potential instability.

## The lateral view

The evaluation of the lateral cervical-spine films should be methodical, and a helpful mnemonic involves the ABCs:

*A stands for alignment, B for bony changes, C for cartilage space, and S for soft tissues.*

The atlas and axis (C1 and C2) need special consideration.

### Alignment

Identify and assess the four lordotic curves on the lateral view of the cervical-spine radiograph (Fig. 11.1). The most anterior curve (a) is a line joining the anterior margins of the cervical vertebral bodies. The second curve (b) is formed by a line drawn along the posterior margins of the cervical vertebral bodies. This line forms the outline of the anterior border of the spinal canal. The posterior border of the canal is outlined by the spinolaminal line (c) which is formed by the anterior margins of the bases of the spinous processes. The fourth lordotic line is drawn along the tips of the spinous processes from C2 to C7 (d).

Constructing these four lines is helpful in assessment of alignment of the vertebrae and in detection of any impingement upon the spinal canal. Each line should form a smooth, continuous, lordotic curve and any disruption suggests a bony or ligamentous injury (an exception to this is the pseudosubluxation of C2 and C3, commonly seen in infants and children, due to immature muscular development with resultant hypermobile spine). When vertebral malalignment of more than 3 mm is present, dislocation must be considered as the normal alignment is usually precise to within 1–2 mm.

The anteroposterior diameter of the spinal canal can be assessed by the space between the lines (b) and (c). This normally measures about 18 mm, and if less than 13 mm, the possibility of spinal-cord compression should be considered.

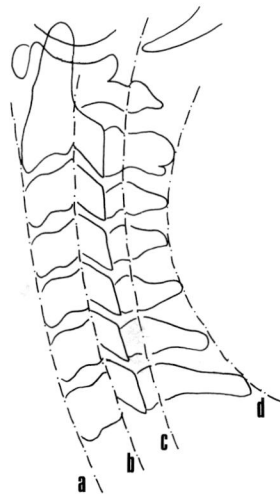

**Fig. 11.1** Cervical spine, lateral view: a, line of anterior bodies; b, line of posterior bodies; c, line of posterior canal; d, line of posterior spinous processes.

### Bone

The contour and height of the vertebral bodies should be assessed. The heights of the anterior and posterior aspects of the vertebral body should be equal for C3–T1. The four corners of each vertebral body must be inspected for fracture lines and avulsions. Osteophytes, ossifications in ligaments, annuli, and ring apophyses can mimic avulsions and can make evaluation of the vertebral margin difficult. The posterior elements should be assessed for signs of disruption or displacement. The articular facets and their supporting pillars appear as a series of nearly quadrilateral structures immediately posterior to the vertebral bodies. They should be evenly spaced and have a slight overlap. In a true lateral view, the left and right pillars will be superimposed and appear as a single structure.

### Cartilage

Assessment should include the intervertebral disc spaces and interspinous spaces. Cartilage space assessment can be used to evaluate the condition of supportive tissues which, when disrupted, may be associated with dislocations. Look for the widening of the intervertebral disc spaces at the anterior and posterior aspect and the interspinous spaces. Slight widening or narrowing of these spaces may be the only clue to an unstable dislocation. Angulation of the interspace of more than 11° when compared with either of the adjacent interspaces suggests clinical instability.

### Soft-tissue spaces

These are:

• the predental space

• the prevertebral spaces

• the prevertebral fat stripe.

Retropharyngeal soft-tissue changes following prevertebral swelling and haemorrhage may be the only radiographic signs in some cases of significant spinal injury. This is especially so for hyperextension injuries which tend to become reduced spontaneously immediately following trauma.

The spaces shown in Table 11.3 should be measured.

*Prevertebral fat stripe*   This is seen as linear lucencies running parallel to the anterior longitudinal ligament. The obliteration of the prevertebral fat stripe is a sign of a fracture at that level. On the other hand, anterior bulging of the prevertebral fat stripe is a indirect sign of an underlying bony or soft-tissue injury.

## The anteroposterior view

It is again important to ensure that the film is adequate, such that C3 to T1 are visible. C1 to C3 may be obscured by the mandible and occiput which overlie them (Fig. 11.2).

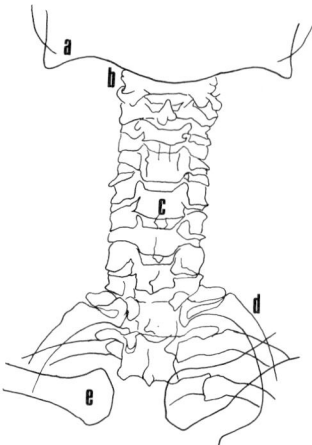

**Fig. 11.2** Cervical spine, frontal view: a, angle of mandible; b, second cervical vertebra; c, spinous process; d, first rib; e, clavicle.

**Table 11.3**  Soft-tissue spaces

| Soft-tissue spaces | Measurements | Remarks |
| --- | --- | --- |
| Predental space | 3 mm or less in adults<br>5 mm or less in children | This is the distance between the anterior aspect of the dens and the posterior aspect of the body of C1. A widening of this space indicates an injury of C1 or C2 |
| Anterior to C2 | 7 mm or less in both children and adults | |
| At C3 and C4 | 5 mm or less | Or it should measure less than half the width of the vertebral body |
| Below C4 | 22 mm or less in adults<br>14 mm or less in children (under 15 years) | The prevertebral soft-tissue space is widened by the presence of the oesophagus and the cricopharyngeal muscles. The retrotracheal space is between the anterior border of the body of C6 to the posterior wall of the trachea<br>In children less than 2 years old the retropharyngeal space appears widened during expiration |

### Alignment

The spinous processes should be in the midline as well as in alignment with each other. The space between each spinous process and the next should be approximately equal.

### Bones, cartilage, and soft tissues

The cortex should be inspected for any steps, breaks, and abnormal angulations. The vertebral bodies should be rectangular and any compression may result in alteration of this shape. The end plates should be inspected for any steps, and the internal trabecular pattern inspected for any alterations or any increase in density which may indicate a possible overlap of bone fragments.

The height of the intervertebral joint spaces should be assessed. The joint space should be similar to that of the adjacent vertebral levels and the articulating surfaces parallel to one another.

## The open-mouth view

The open-mouth view shows the C1/C2 articulation (Fig. 11.3).

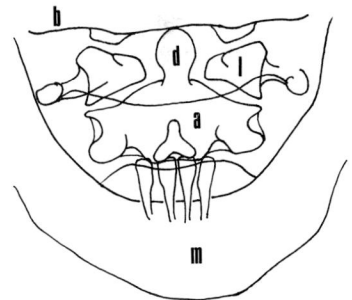

**Fig. 11.3**  Odontoid peg, open-mouth view: a, axis; b, base of skull; l, lateral mass of atlas; m, mandible. The space between the odontoid peg and the lateral mass of the atlas should be symmetrical and equidistant on both sides.

*Alignment*

Ensure that the odontoid peg (dens) and spinous process of C2 lie in the same vertical line and that the lateral masses of C1 and C2 are in alignment. The space between the lateral masses of the atlas and the odontoid peg should be symmetrical. Jefferson fractures and rotatory subluxation of the odontoid in children are also best shown by the open-mouth view.

*Bones*

Assess the odontoid peg for evidence of fractures, either of the peg itself, at the base, or into the body of C2. The shadow of some structures that can be mistaken for fractures include overlying teeth, the occiput, and the epiphyseal plate. Fusion of the epiphysis normally occurs at 12 years of age, but if union does not occur, an os odontoideum may be seen at the tip of the peg.

*Cartilage and soft tissues*

The articulating surfaces should be parallel to one another. Soft-tissue shadows in general are not assessed in this view.

## Injuries involving the atlas–axis

Injuries involving C1 and C2 are sometimes difficult to assess because of the following factors:

1. Coexisting head injury with altered conscious level may result in the absence of a history of the mechanism of injury, and the lack of physical signs of injury.

2. The low incidence of accompanying neurological sequelae at this level in blunt trauma survivors decreases the level of suspicion.

3. The overlap of bony structures and spondylosis

4. Some fracture lines may be difficult to detect on routine radiography if they are oblique to the radiographic beam.

However, indirect evidence of injury may present itself in the radiological clues listed in Table 11.4.

## The oblique views

These show the posterior elements of the vertebrae, including the neural foraminae and the facet joints. They may be performed without moving the patient, by angling the tube.

## The flexion and extension views

These views are reserved for patients with abnormal alignment and suspicion of injuries to soft tissues supporting the vertebrae which are

**Table 11.4**  Clues to injury involving the atlas–axis

| Radiological abnormality | Injuries |
| --- | --- |
| Displacement of the articular masses of C1 on the open-mouth view | Disruption of the ring of the atlas, or transverse ligament and/or alar ligament injury |
| Increase of the interspinous distance of C1 and C2 | Posterior ligamentous disruption and possible fractures of anterior elements |
| Displacement of the spinous process of C2 of more than 2 mm behind the posterior spinous process line | Hangman's fracture |
| Soft-tissue swelling | Injury to blood vessels close to the damaged ligamentous structures |
| A predental space width of more than 5 mm in a child or 3 mm in an adult | Injury to the C1 or C2 |

not obvious on the standard radiographs. It must be remembered that the flexion and extension views are done to demonstrate instability and therefore it is imperative that only voluntary flexion and extension by the patient is allowed and should not be forced. It should be done in the presence of a doctor who is qualified to supervise a patient with an unstable cervical spine. These views should be examined as described earlier using the ABCs system.

# IMAGING OF SPECIFIC CERVICAL-SPINE INJURIES

The mechanism and types of cervical-spine injury are summarized in Table 11.5.

## Jefferson fractures

This is a burst fracture of the C1 vertebra. The injury usually results from axial loading and compression of the C1 ring (Figs 11.4, 11.5).

This injury is unstable but is uncommon for neurological symptoms to occur as the fragments are displaced laterally away from the cord.

Burst fractures involving the lower cervical levels are more likely to be symptomatic and predispose to cord damage. Fragments that are displaced posteriorly are likely to cause cord damage as the spinal canal at lower levels is not as capacious as at the C1 and C2 level.

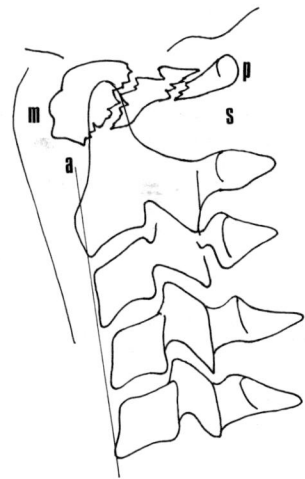

**Fig. 11.4**  Cervical spine, lateral view, Jefferson fracture: a, disruption of the anterior line; m, prevertebral haematoma—widening of the precervical vertebral soft tissue; p, posterior fragments; s, widened interspinous distance.

**Table 11.5**   Mechanism of cervical-spine injuries and the types of injury

| Mechanism | Types of injury |
| --- | --- |
| Flexion | Anterior subluxation<br>Bilateral facet joint dislocation<br>Simple wedge fracture<br>Clay shoveller's fracture<br>Teardrop fracture |
| Flexion and rotation | Unilateral facet joint dislocation |
| Hyperextension | Avulsion fracture of anterior arch of atlas<br>Extension teardrop fracture<br>Fracture of posterior arch of atlas<br>Laminar fracture<br>Hangman's fracture |
| Hyperextension and rotation | Pillar fracture<br>Fracture separation of the lateral mass |
| Compression | Jefferson fracture (C1 vertebra)<br>Burst fracture |

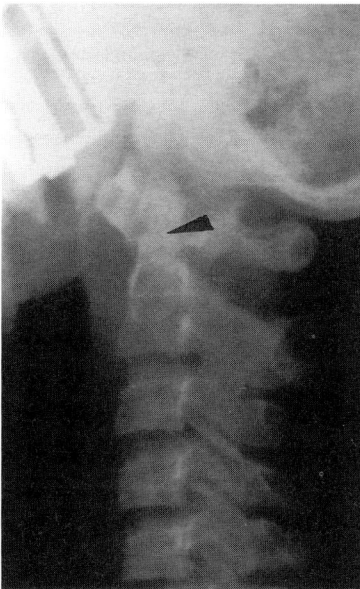

**Fig. 11.5**   Open-mouth view, Jefferson fracture: *, lateral displacement of the lateral mass of atlas with widening of the ipsilateral space between the odontoid peg and the lateral mass of atlas.

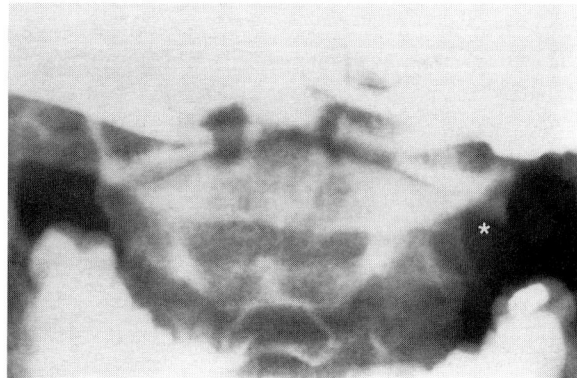

**Fig. 11.6**   Cervical spine, lateral view, odontoid peg fracture: ◄, anterior displacement of the fractured odontoid peg.

## Odontoid fractures

This should be carefully looked for on the lateral and open-mouth views. The commonly involved area is at the junction of the odontoid peg and the body of the C2 vertebra (type 2) and through the upper body of a vertebra (type 3). On the lateral view, there is usually a loss of continuity between the anterior cortical margin of the C2 body and the peg (Figs 11.6, 11.7).

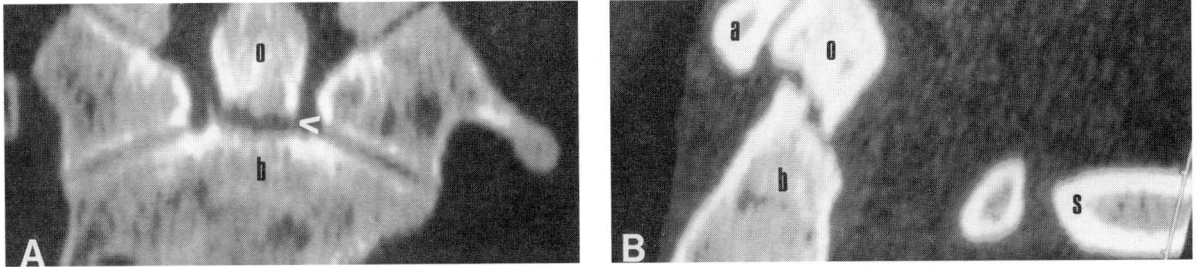

**Fig. 11.7** CT cervical spine (atlas and axis), odontoid peg fracture. (A) Coronal reconstruction; (B) sagittal reconstruction. **V,** Fracture line seen clearly across the base of the odontoid peg; a, anterior arch of atlas; b, body of axis; o, odontoid peg; s, spinous process.

## Hangman's fracture

This is a fracture involving the pedicles and pars interarticularis of C2 with an associated traumatic spondylolisthesis (Fig. 11.8, 11.9). It should be treated as unstable. The mechanism is usually a combination of hyperextension and axial compression, as may occur in diving and rugby accidents.

## Facet joint dislocation

### Bilateral facet dislocation

Anterior subluxation due to bilateral facet dislocation is an extremely serious injury with a high incidence of spinal-cord damage. Radiologically there is anterolisthesis slip of 50 per cent or more on the lateral view (Fig. 11.10). This injury is usually due to flexion.

### Unilateral facet dislocation

This is an important injury, resulting from flexion–rotation injury. The most commonly affected areas are the C4–C6 vertebrae. Radiologically, there is anterior subluxation which is less than half of the vertebral body width, with the dislocated facet positioned anteriorly (Fig. 11.11). There is also widening of the soft tissues anteriorly. On the anteroposterior views, the spinous process is rotated to the side of dislocation.

## Teardrop fracture–dislocation

One mechanism of this injury is due to axial loading and flexion. It is markedly unstable and potentially life threatening. The lower cervical spine is commonly involved. Radiologically, a small triangular

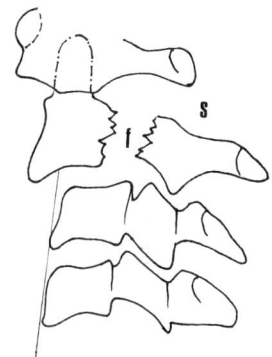

**Fig. 11.8** Cervical spine, lateral view, hangman's fracture: f, fracture of the axis (second cervical vertebra) pedicles; s, widening of the interspinous distance.

fragment of the anteroinferior margin of one of the cervical vertebrae is seen (Fig. 11.12). Complete ligamentous disruption may accompany this injury, resulting in subluxation and cord compression.

The other mechanism that produces this injury is hyperextension, which results in the rupture of the anterior longitudinal ligament with a typical triangular fragment. These fractures occur more often in older, osteoporotic patients with spondylosis. Prevertebral soft-tissue swelling is frequently present. This injury is unstable (Figs 11.14 and 11.15).

## Other flexion injuries

Most structural flexion injuries of the cervical spine are extremely unstable. However, some flexion–compression fractures may not be associated with significant neurological symptoms. One such example is the clay shoveller's fracture, an oblique avulsion injury of the spinous process (Fig. 11.13), which can occur without significant sequelae. This injury usually involves the spinous processes of C6, C7, or T1. Ligamentous injuries may also be present in cases of hyperflexion injury and, in these instances, upright lateral, flexion, and extension views may be necessary.

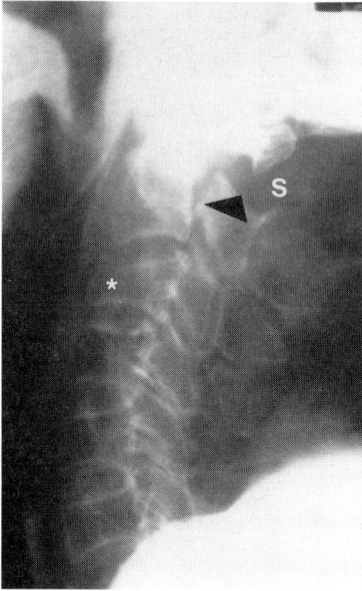

**Fig. 11.9** Cervical spine, lateral view, hangman's fracture: * compression fracture of the third vertebral body; ◄, fracture of the second cervical vertebral pedicles; s, widening of the interspinous distance between the first and second vertebral spinous processes.

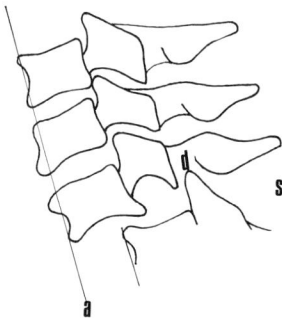

**Fig. 11.10** Cervical spine, lateral view, bilateral facet dislocation: a, anterior displacement of cephalad vertebral bodies; d, dislocated facets; s, widened interspinous distance.

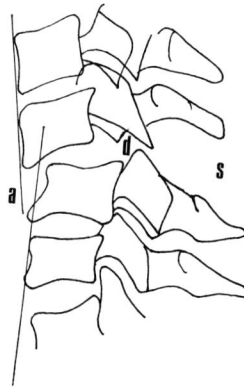

**Fig. 11.11** Cervical spine, lateral view, unilateral facet dislocation: a, anterior displacement of cephalad vertebral bodies of less than half of one vertebral body width; d, superior facet forward dislocation; s, widened interspinous distance.

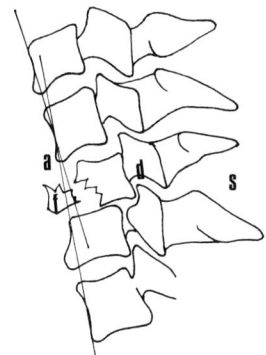

**Fig. 11.12** Cervical spine, lateral view, flexion teardrop fracture dislocation: a, anterior angulation at the fracture site; d, subluxed facet; f, fracture fragment; s, widened interspinous distance.

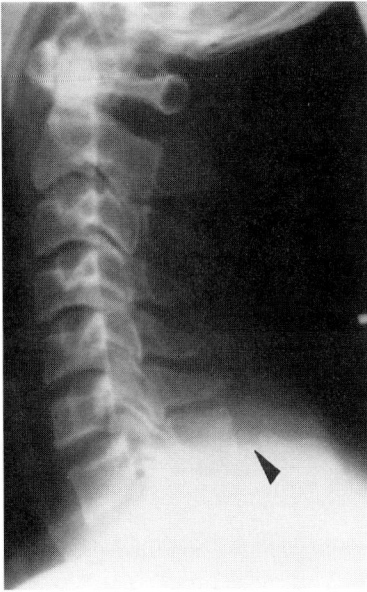

**Fig. 11.13** Cervical spine, lateral view: ◄, avulsion fracture of the seventh cervical vertebral spinous process.

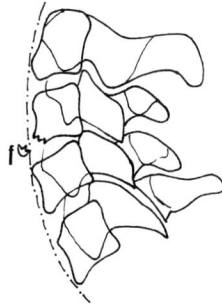

**Fig. 11.14** Cervical spine, lateral view, extension teardrop fracture: f, fracture fragment from the anteroinferior end plate of the vertebral body.

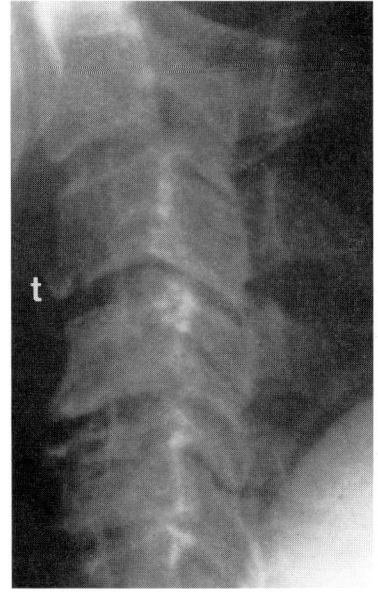

**Fig. 11.15** Cervical spine, lateral view, extension teardrop fracture: t, fracture fragment.

## Hyperextension injuries

Hyperextension of the cervical spine places the most stress on the posterior elements. This may lead to fractures of the posterior ring and spinous process. All posterior fractures should be treated as unstable injuries. When hyperextension occurs in combination with rotation, the resultant fractures include pillar fractures and fracture separation of the lateral mass. Pillar fracture results from impaction of the articulating mass by the ipsilateral superior articular mass during hyperextension and rotation. In fracture separation of the lateral mass, the pedicle and lamina fracture at the junction with the lateral mass. The lateral mass is separated from the vertebral body and lamina and is free-floating.

## Cervical-spine injuries in children

Although there is more elasticity in a child's vertebral column, which increases the vulnerability of the spine to traumatic forces, cervical-spine injuries are less common in children than in adults. There are also some differences between the anatomy of children and adults.

**Differences between the paediatric and adult cervical spine**

Differences in the head and neck:

1.  Size of the head. Children have a relatively bigger head, which may result in a greater incidence of flexion–extension injuries due to the greater angular momentum that is generated in accidents.

2.  Smaller neck muscle mass. The incidence of ligamentous injuries is higher than that of fractures due to the poor protection offered by the smaller muscle mass.

Differences in the bones and ligaments:

1.  Interspinous ligaments and joint capsules are more flexible.

2.  Facet joints are flatter and have a more horizontal orientation.

3.  Uncinate articulations are less developed.

4.  Vertebral bodies are biconcave in shape with slight anterior wedging. This may give the false impression of possible compression fractures.

Differences in the soft-tissue spaces:

1.  Increased preodontoid space. This is seen in 20 per cent of younger children.

2.  Widening of the prevertebral spaces. The prevertebral spaces are more difficult to evaluate in children as variations occur during respiration (increased retropharyngeal space during expiration and crying), neck positioning, and increased mass of retropharyngeal lymph nodes.

Developmental differences:

1.  Incomplete ossification. Interpretation of the bony alignment may be difficult and may give a false impression of possible fracture lines. Fusion of the basilar odontoid synchondrosis occurs between 3 and 7 years of age. The apical odontoid epiphyseal tip may be mistaken for a fracture. Fusion of the posterior arch of C1 occurs by 4 years of age and the anterior arch between 7 and 10 years of age.

2.  Pseudosubluxation of C2 and C3. This is a normal variant in up to 40 per cent of children less than 7 years of age and is due to increased ligamentous laxity. It is present in under 20 per cent of those aged 7–16 years. Displacement may be up to 3 mm anteriorly. Pseudosubluxation of C3 on C4 occurs less commonly.

An algorithm for the evaluation of patients with suspected cervical-spine injuries is shown in Fig. 11.16.

Possible CERVICAL-SPINE INJURIES

↓

Cross-table lateral radiograph

↓

Is the C7–T1 junction adequately visualized ?

Yes　　　　　　　　　No

Normal　　　Abnormal　　　Swimmer's view or lateral
view with traction on
arms

↓

Other views: A–P　　Further evaluation　　If C7–T1 junction still not
and open-mouth if　　with CT or MRI　　visualized or suspicious
condition allows　　while maintaining　　of abnormality
　　　　　　　　　　C spine
　　　　　　　　　　immobilization

Normal　　Suspicious　　　　　　　CT of the area (C7–T1)
　　　　　of injury

Stop　　　1. MRI　　　　Abnormal　　　Normal
further　　2. Flexion
investigation　　extension　　　　　　Complete the
　　　　　views*　　　　　　　　　rest of
　　　　　　　　　　　　　　　　cervical series

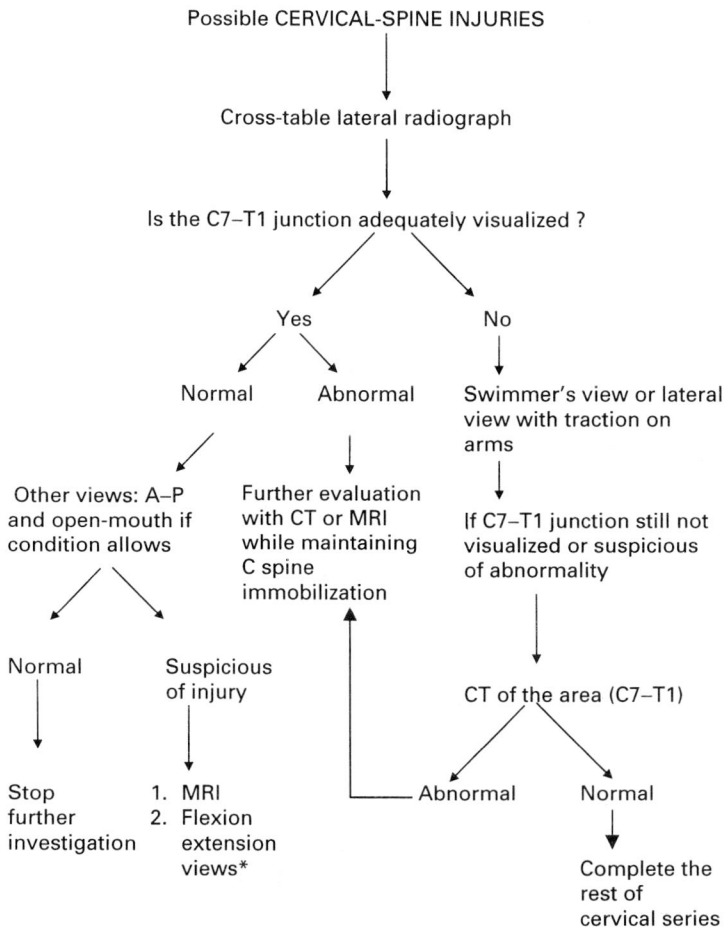

**Fig. 11.16** Algorithm for the evaluation of patients with suspected cervical spine injuries.
* To be performed under medical supervision.

## SOFT-TISSUE INJURIES

Although the neck is protected to a certain extent, superiorly by the face and inferiorly by the chest, it is still an area vulnerable to injuries from both blunt and penetrating trauma.

### Blunt trauma to the neck

Patients who sustain blunt trauma to the neck may be victims of major trauma and may have sustained other injuries as well. In those who have injuries localized to the neck, the mechanisms include kick and punch, and assault with blunt objects such as baseball bats and metal pipes. Accompanying significant soft-tissue swelling and haematoma formation may compromise the airway, particularly in those patients with laryngeal fractures. The possible involvement of the cervical spine, and hence its stability, must also be considered.

Blunt injuries to the vascular, visceral, and neural elements may occur. Injuries to the brachiocephalic arteries can occur in combination with aortic injuries in the chest, and blunt vascular injuries may cause neurological deficits that are characteristically delayed in onset.

## Penetrating neck trauma

The majority of penetrating neck wounds are caused by stabbing and, less commonly, by gunshot injuries. The majority of life-threatening injuries caused by penetrating injury are vascular, presenting either as massive or occult haemorrhage. Occult haemorrhage can remain asymptomatic for some time, as for example bleeding from the carotid artery which is limited by the carotid sheath.

Nerves are frequently involved but any neurological deficits may not be due solely to direct nerve injuries. Vascular injury may impair the blood supply to the brain and a number of major neural structures in the neck.

Injuries to the aerodigestive tract may not be apparent on initial presentation, especially when other associated critical injuries are also present. The risk of injuries to the vascular system, respiratory passages, digestive tract, and nervous system warrants surgical exploration of most penetrating neck wounds. In addition, wound exploration is indicated when evaluation is difficult, as in patients who are under the influence of alcohol or drugs.

## THE TECHNIQUES AVAILABLE FOR IMAGING SOFT-TISSUE INJURIES

### Conventional radiography

While a standard cross-table lateral radiograph of the neck is mandatory (refer to cervical-spine injuries) for most patients with deceleration injuries, soft-tissue techniques should be employed if there is any suspicion of airway injury as these enable better airway and precervi-

**Table 11.6** Conventional radiography of the neck

| Signs | Injuries indicated |
| --- | --- |
| Lateral neck radiographs | |
|   Free air in the soft tissues | Rupture of the oesophagus or trachea |
|   Displacement of air column | Soft-tissue masses, swelling, or haematoma |
|   ABCs* abnormalities | Cervical-spine injuries with or without cord injuries |
|   Foreign bodies, bullet(s), or missile fragments | Penetrating injuries with retained foreign bodies confirmed |
| Anteroposterior neck radiographs | |
|   Abnormal shape of hyoid bone | Hyoid bone fracture |
| Chest radiographs | |
|   Pneumothorax, pneumomediastinum, haemothorax | Tracheal, oesophageal, great vessel, or aortic injuries |
|   Any foreign bodies or bullet or missile fragment | Penetrating injuries with retained foreign bodies confirmed |

* Alignment, Bones, Cartilage, and Soft tissues.

cal soft-tissue evaluation (Fig. 11.17). In penetrating injuries, foreign bodies (including bullets and pellets from gunshot injuries) can be localized.

As the root of the neck is in direct connection with the chest, coexisting chest injuries are not uncommon in both blunt and penetrating mechanisms. A chest radiograph is essential for the evaluation of associated chest injuries, such as pneumothorax, haemothorax, or pneumomediastinum.

Table 11.6 summarizes the injuries that may be indicated by conventional radiography.

## Computed tomography

CT is especially valuable in the evaluation of the airway after blunt trauma. In most injuries, it is able to define the type and degree of injury of both soft tissue and bone.

It must be emphasized that although there may be a pressing need to evaluate the airway, investigations should not be attempted in a patient who is at risk of sudden deterioration as a result of an acute airway injury. The priority in this case would be to secure and maintain a patent airway first before sending the patient for scanning.

In stable patients MRI is undoubtedly best for the evaluation of soft-tissue injuries of the neck, but its limitations in the acute situation have been mentioned earlier. Fortunately, CT is able to

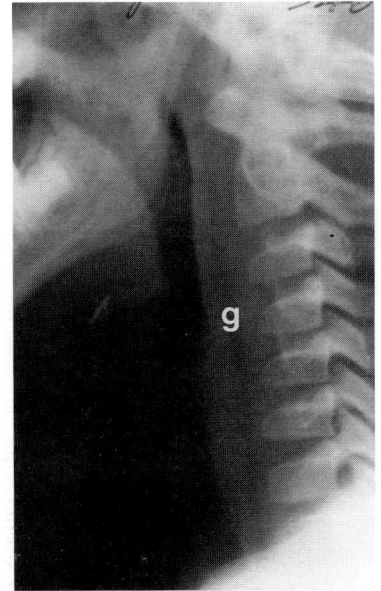

**Fig. 11.17** Neck, lateral view: g, precervical soft-tissue gas due to mucosal tear as a result of laryngeal trauma.

demonstrate soft-tissue and bony injuries of the neck satisfactorily in most of the cases.

## Angiography

One of the challenges in the management of neck injuries is the diagnosis of asymptomatic vascular injuries. If vascular injuries are not diagnosed early, they are frequently associated with high morbidity and sometimes mortality. Angiography remains the investigation of choice in the evaluation of vascular injuries and serves as a guide in planning the operative treatment.

When considering vascular injuries in penetrating neck trauma, it is helpful to separate the neck wounds according to the three zones (Table 11.1). This division has a bearing on the patient's management. Performing angiography is considered the standard approach by many trauma surgeons for penetrating injuries in zones I and III. In symptomatic injuries to zone II, exploration and repair can be performed readily without the need for angiography. In zone III injuries, angiography is usually required to assess the status of both the internal carotid arteries and the intracranial circulation.

A complete angiographic study would include a four-vessel examination, imaging each of the carotid and vertebral arteries with intracranial views.

In addition to its diagnostic role, angiography also has a therapeutic role in the management of vascular injuries of the neck. It allows embolization, for instance, of a traumatic aneurysm when a direct surgical approach is difficult or not possible.

## Other studies

### Fibreoptic endoscopy

In appropriate patients, fibreoptic endoscopy examinations of the gastrointestinal and respiratory tracts have proved useful for the evaluation of injuries to these structures.

### Gastrograffin oesophagrams

Suspected oesophageal injuries, such as a tear or rupture, may be evaluated by the use of gastrograffin oesophagrams. However, this technique has a high false-negative rate of up to 25 per cent. Therefore only positive findings are helpful, and constant clinical review of the patient would be required in those with a negative study.

BLUNT NECK INJURY

↓

Airway assessment + cervical spine immobilization

Patent airway                    Obstructed airway

↓                                ↓

Supplemental oxygen          Endotracheal intubation
by facial mask                or surgical airway

↓

Assessment of other injuries
and underlying structures of the neck for signs of injury

↓

Appropriate baseline blood investigation;
radiological examination
(cross lateral C spine, CXR and pelvic X-ray*)

| Laryngeal or tracheal injury | Oesophageal injury | Vascular injury | Cervical-spine injury |

Assess vital signs and worsening of clinical symptoms repeatedly

Assess vital signs and clinical observation

Assess vital signs and neurological status repeatedly**

Cervical-spine immobilization and assess neurological status

Diagnostic modalities:
Laryngoscopy
Endoscopy
CT scan
Brochoscopy

Diagnostic modalities:
Oesophagography
Oesophagoscopy

Refer to Figure 11.16

Stable condition          Unstable condition

Definitive airway management

Arteriography

Immediate surgical intervention

Admit for observation and surgical intervention

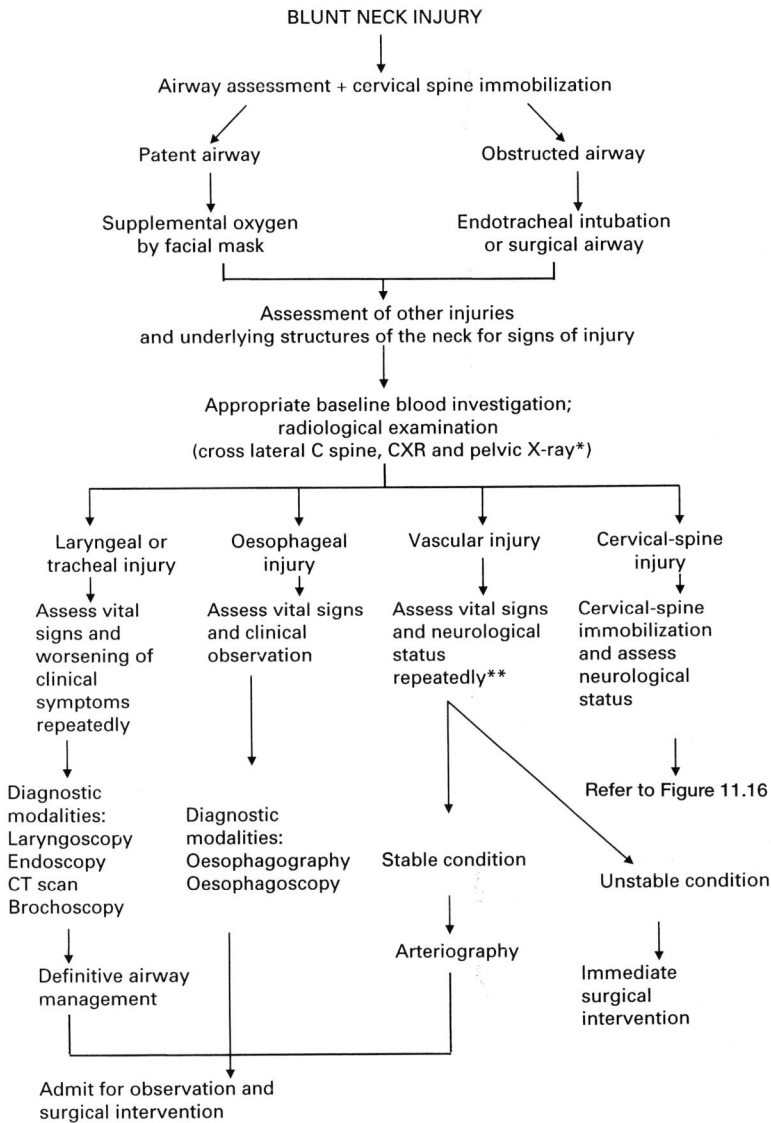

**Fig. 11.18** Algorithm for the evaluation of patients with a blunt neck injury. *, Pelvic X-ray indicated in multiple trauma patients; **, neurological deficit occurs in vascular injuries.

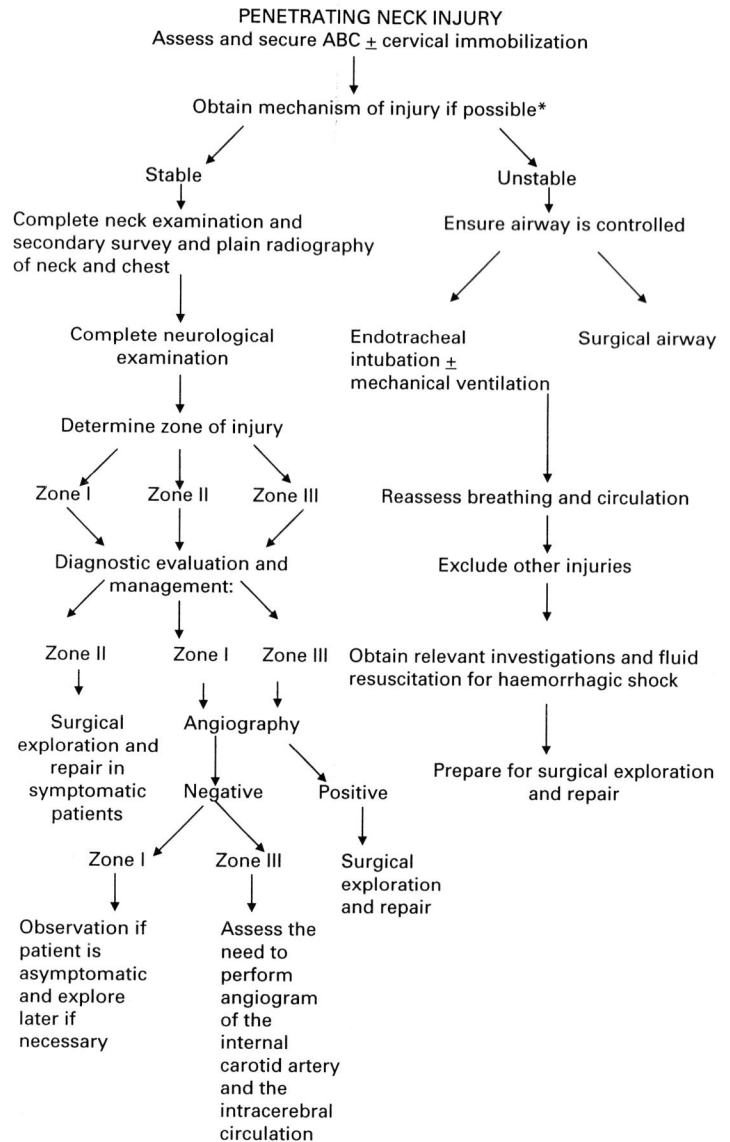

**Fig. 11.19** Algorithm for evaluation of penetrating neck injuries. *, Mechanism of injury: stab wounds by knives; gunshots; motor vehicles; or industrial accidents. Note: stab wounds tend to involve the left side and are accompanied by external bleeding, and gunshot wounds penetrate deeply and more commonly produce serious bleeding and haematomas in the neck.

Algorithms for the evaluation of patients with blunt and penetrating neck injuries are shown in Figs 11.18 and 11.19, respectively.

# BIBLIOGRAPHY

Allen BL, Ferguson RL, Lehman TR, *et al*. A mechanistic classification of closed, indirect fractures and dislocations of the lower cervical spine. Spine 1982; 7:1–27.

Ballinger PW. Merrill's Atlas of Radiographic Positions and Radiologic Procedures, 8th edn. Missouri: Mosby 1995; 2:11–28.

Beatson TR. Fractures and dislocations of the cervical spine. J Bone Joint Surg (Br) 1963; 45:21–35.

Berquist TH, Cabonela ME. In: Berquist TH, ed. The Spine Imaging of Orthopaedic Trauma and Surgery. Philadelphia: WB Saunders, 1986.

Cattell HS, Filtzer DL. Pseudosubluxation and other normal variations of the cervical spine of children. J Bone Joint Surg 1965; 47(A):1295.

Daffner RH. Imaging of Vertebral Trauma. Rockville, MD: Aspen, 1988.

Denis F. Spinal instability as defined by the three column spine concept in acute spinal trauma. Clin Orthop 1984; 189:65–76.

Dosch JC. Trauma: Conventional Radiological Study in Spine Injury. Berlin: Springer-Verlag, 1985.

Fielding JW, Hawkins RJ. Roentgen diagnosis of the injured neck. Instr Course Lect 1976; 25:149–70.

Gehweiler JA Jr, Clark WM, Schaff RE, *et al*. Cervical spine trauma: the common combined conditions. Radiology 1979; 130:77–86.

Gehweiler JA, Osborne RL, Becker RF. The Radiology of Vertebral Trauma. Philadelphia: WB Saunders, 1980.

Harris JH, Edeiken MB, eds. The Radiology of Acute Cervical Spine Trauma, 2nd edn. Baltimore: Williams & Wilkins, 1987; 119–21.

Harris JH Jr, Yeakley JS. Radiologically subtle soft tissue injuries of the cervical spine. Curr Probl Diagn Radiol 1989; 25:167–90.

Holdsworth FW. Fractures, dislocations and fracture dislocations of the spine. J Bone Joint Surg 1970; 52A:1534–51.

Meschan IA. An Atlas of Anatomy Basic to Radiology. Philadelphia: WB Saunders, 1975.

Rogers LF. Radiology of Skeletal Trauma. New York: Churchill Livingstone, 1982.

Swischuk LE. Anterior dislocation of C2 in children: physiologic or pathologic. Radiology 1977; 122:759.

Tarr RW, Drolshagagen LF, Kerner TC, *et al*. MR imaging of recent spinal trauma. J Comput Assist Tomogr 1987; 11:412–19.

Weir DC. Roentgenographic signs of cervical injury. Clin Orthop 1975; 109:9–17.

# CHAPTER 12

# *The chest*

........................................................................................................................................................................

- Key points: the chest
- Clinical anatomy
- Evaluation
- The techniques available
- Imaging of specific conditions
- Bibliography

## Key points: the chest

1. Injuries to the abdominal organs should be suspected if chest injuries that occur below the nipple line are discovered.

2. The likelihood of injury to the various organs can be predicted by the mechanism of injury and be proactively sought.

3. It may not possible to perform an erect chest radiograph in a posteroanterior projection in trauma victims. When interpreting a supine anteroposterior view, the limitations and differences in appearance of this projection must be taken into account.

4. Do not focus in too closely when interpreting a chest radiograph, as abnormalities are likely to be spotted more easily from a few feet away.

5. Chest radiographs should not be performed solely to diagnose rib fractures, but rather to detect complications and associated underlying pleural or pulmonary injuries suspected on clinical examination.

6. Ultrasonography is valuable for the bedside emergency evaluation of cardiac trauma.

7. Although conventional radiography provides sufficient information for most chest injuries, computed tomography provides additional information that helps in subsequent patient management.

## CLINICAL ANATOMY

The chest can be divided arbitrarily into the bony framework—the thoracic cage—and the organs and structures lying within it. The thoracic cage is formed by the vertebral column posteriorly, the ribs and intercostal spaces on either side, and the sternum and costal cartilages in front. Superiorly, the sternum articulates with the clavicle and first ribs and forms the thoracic inlet, which communicates with the root of the neck. Inferiorly, it is separated from the abdominal cavity by the diaphragm.

## The bony thoracic cage

The sternum is made up of the manubrium, body, and the xiphoid process. The sternal angle is the junction between the body of the sternum and the manubrium. The sternum overlies the heart and mediastinal contents, and serves as a partial external protector of these structures. However, fractures involving the sternum with backward displacement may result in injuries to the heart. The attachment of the sternum to the elastic costal cartilages protects it to some extent from injuries, but the elasticity reduces with advancing age, and calcification commonly occurs, which can be seen on radiographs.

The greater part of the thoracic cage is formed by the 12 pairs of ribs. Of these, the first seven pairs are connected anteriorly by the costal cartilages to the sternum; the cartilages of the eighth, ninth, and tenth ribs each articulate with the cartilage of the rib above; and the last two ribs are free laterally. The ribs may be fractured by direct force, or indirectly by compressive injuries and bending stresses. In compressive injuries to the chest, ribs tend to fracture at their angle, which is the weakest part. The upper two ribs, which are protected by the clavicle, and the lower two ribs, which are free, are the least commonly injured. In severe crush injuries to the chest, several ribs may fracture at more than one point so that a whole segment of the thoracic cage becomes detached from the rest of the chest wall. This is termed a flail segment and may move paradoxically with respiration.

In children, the chest wall is highly elastic and therefore fractures of the ribs are uncommon, even in the presence of serious injuries to the underlying organs and soft tissues.

## The pleura

In normal circumstances, the pleural membranes do not cast a significant radiographic shadow except at the costophrenic angles, where a minimal shadow is seen. The parietal and visceral pleural layers are in close apposition and the space between them is only a potential one and therefore not seen radiographically. In pneumothorax, the separation can be seen, with air between the two layers. Normally, the costophrenic angles are sharply delineated and the presence of blunting to any significant degree is due either to previous pleural disease or new fluid accumulation.

## The diaphragm

The diaphragm divides the thoracic from the abdominal cavity and is pierced by the following structures: the superior epigastric artery, musculophrenic artery, the splanchnic nerves and the sympathetic trunks posteriorly, aorta, azygos vein, thoracic duct passing between the crura, the inferior vena cava, oesophagus, and two vagus nerves. On quiet breathing, the vertical range of movement of the diaphragm is about 1–2 cm and this increases to 3–5 cm on deep breathing. Therefore, injuries to the chest may involve the abdominal cavity and vice versa.

## The mediastinum

The mediastinum is bounded laterally by the reflections of the parietal pleura of the medial aspects of both lungs. Superiorly, it is bounded by the thoracic inlet and inferiorly by the diaphragm. The posterior aspect of the sternum forms the anterior border and the posterior boundary is formed by anterior surfaces of the thoracic vertebral bodies. The mediastinum is divided arbitrarily for descriptive purposes. A line drawn from the sternal angle to the intervertebral space between the T4 and T5 vertebrae divides it into superior and inferior mediastinum anterior to the pericardium, a middle mediastinum containing the heart and the great vessels, and the posterior mediastinum between the posterior aspect of the heart and the lower eight thoracic vertebrae. Any injuries to the mediastinal structures may be reflected radiologically in changes in the size and shape of the mediastinum.

## The heart and great vessels

The mediastinal and cardiac shadows may vary in shape and size in patients with different build. In asthenic (tall, thin) people, the mediastinum as a whole is long and narrow. The diaphragm is low and the cardiac shadow tends to be long, narrow and rather straight up and down. The pulmonary shadow tends to be rather prominent. In the pyknic patient (short, broad), the mediastinal shadow tends to be shorter and wider on the whole. The diaphragm is high and the cardiac contours tend to be markedly convex.

The cardiac silhouette changes in shape on changing the body position. The change from the erect to the recumbent position causes a broadening of the cardiac silhouette, especially at its base. In pregnant patients, the diaphragm is elevated and the lungs show an apparent increased vascularity, resulting from enlargement of the breasts causing an increased haziness at both lung bases.

# EVALUATION

In the evaluation of chest trauma, it is important to remember that injuries to one thoracic organ may affect the others, as the functions of the heart and lung are closely related in achieving full oxygenation of the tissues and organs of the other parts of the body.

Any injuries below the nipple level should alert the physician to the possibility of coexisting abdominal injuries, as the diaphragm rises to that level during full expiration, and the length of many weapons causing penetrating injury would easily allow diaphragmatic penetration.

The mechanism of injury is especially important in the determination of the likelihood of injuries to the various organs. In blunt chest trauma, the chest wall has the highest likelihood of being injured (rib fractures and flail chest) with secondary risks of pneumothorax, haemothorax, and lung contusion. In penetrating chest trauma, the risks of direct pulmonary, cardiac, and diaphragmatic injuries are increased.

## Blunt chest trauma

Most blunt chest trauma results from motor vehicle accidents (80 per cent), falls with a blow to the chest, and industrial accidents. Of patients with blunt chest injuries who arrive alive at the hospital, only a minority die of isolated chest injuries (3 per cent). The same percentage die from associated head injuries, and another 2 per cent from other causes, including mostly abdominal injuries.

Initial treatment of major injuries should follow the usual guidelines: airway, breathing, and circulation. As discussed in Chapter 5, the following specific injuries can kill within a short time and should be identified and appropriate treatment instituted immediately: flail chest, tension pneumothorax, open pneumothorax, massive haemothorax, and cardiac tamponade.

Multiple rib fractures and flail chest may cause great pain, and commonly result in hypoxia requiring respiratory support. This may be compounded by haemothorax and pneumothorax which are often also present. A pneumothorax that continues to leak actively, or fails to resolve, indicates a possible ruptured bronchus and requires further diagnostic work-up. Massive haemothorax (defined as an initial chest drain output greater than 1200 ml or continued bleeding at a rate of 200 ml/h for three consecutive hours) is indicative of the need for further investigation and usually emergency thoracotomy. Common causes include torn intercostal vessels, followed by lung or pulmonary vessel injury. Although pneumomediastinum is a spectacular finding, it is usually not lethal and can be considered harmless if significant injuries to the airway and oesophageal injury can be ruled out. It often results from rupture of alveoli deep in the lung, with dissection of air proximally.

## Penetrating chest injuries

The majority of instances of penetrating chest trauma can be managed conservatively by the insertion of a chest drain without operative treatment, as the most common injuries are to the pleura and lungs, which may seal spontaneously. Injuries to the heart and great vessels require surgery in most instances. Penetrating wounds that show evidence of involving the abdominal cavity require exploratory laparotomy. In patients with gunshot wounds to the chest, the damage may be more extensive if the missile traverses the mediastinum from side to side.

# THE TECHNIQUES AVAILABLE

## Conventional radiography

### Chest radiograph: P-A projection

Ideally, the radiographic examination of the chest should be made with the patient in an erect position, using the posteroanterior projection, because physiological alterations of intrathoracic structures may simulate organic disease on the supine radiograph. However, in most instances, in the seriously injured patient, the only examination possible is the supine anteroposterior view.

In patients who are able to assume an erect position, the routine radiographic study of the adult chest should consist of an erect posteroanterior (P-A) film made in deep inspiration. Depending on the mechanism and clinical findings, a lateral projection enables the diagnosis of sternal fractures, which may have important implications in subsequent patient management. In clinical situations when it is impossible to obtain an erect P-A projection, an erect anteroposterior projection is preferable to a supine examination, but neither may be appropriate in the multiple trauma patient when spinal protection is the initial priority.

## Adequacy of projection

When evaluating the lung fields, it is important to have an adequate inspiration as an expiratory film shows increased lung markings which mimic pathological processes. The small, abnormally dense lungs, an enlarged heart, and engorged vascular markings can be mistaken for congestive heart failure if incomplete expansion is not recognized. In general, for an adult an adequate degree of inspiration may be assumed when the posterior part of the right ninth rib is visible above the diaphragmatic surface in the P-A chest radiograph. In infants and children, deep inspiration in chest radiographs is particularly important because in expiration the poorly aerated lung produces a radiographic appearance that closely resembles pneumonia.

The following are features of a good normal chest radiograph:

(1)  a trachea that is situated in the midline;

(2)  a central and symmetrical location of the medial borders of the clavicles over the superior mediastinum;

(3)  equally dense lung fields with symmetrical vascular markings which should be traceable to just 1–2 cm of the chest wall throughout the lungs;

(4)  equally dense pulmonary hila, with the left hilum usually 2 cm higher than the right;

(5)  a mediastinum that is central and has a sharp silhouette;

(6)  the position of the heart shadow is such that one-third of its diameter is to the right and two-thirds is to the left of the spinous processes;

(7)  a cardiothoracic ratio of less than 50 per cent;

(8)  a thoracic spine outline which is just visible through the mediastinum;

(9)  the ribs are visible behind the cardiac shadow with no irregularity in their course or edges;

(10)  well-defined borders of the hemidiaphragms with sharp costophrenic and cardiophrenic angles;

(11)    the dome of the right hemidiaphragm being 0.5–2.5 cm above the left.

The principles involved in the interpretation of the chest radiographs are those applicable to all radiographic examinations, and include evaluating the film systematically. Although it is normally acceptable to look first to the areas of obvious or expected abnormalities, the entire radiograph must also be examined so that important information is not overlooked. A common mistake is to focus in on the film too closely. Important abnormalities may be more easily spotted from a distance of a few feet.

## Anteroposterior (supine) view

In the presence of major trauma the radiographic examination of the chest can only be obtained in the supine position. The mediastinum is wider in this view than in the erect chest examination and the cardiac silhouette increases its transverse diameter. This results from magnification differences and normal increases in mediastinal venous dilatation. Although the superior mediastinum is wider, its margins remain distinct and normal anatomical landmarks are identifiable. Therefore, in the supine examination, mediastinal widening alone does not indicate mediastinal haematoma in the setting of chest trauma. One of the diagnostic limitations when interpreting the supine chest radiograph is in the diagnosis of small pneumothoraces and haemothoraces.

Small or even moderate haemothoraces are not easily discernible. They may appear as increased haziness as the fluid is spread out in the posterior pleural space in recumbency. Pneumothoraces may be impossible to detect because of air migration into the anterior (uppermost) pleural space in a supine patient. If confirmation is needed for a patient who cannot be sat up for an erect examination, a lateral decubitus examination of the chest may be taken with the side of suspected pneumothorax up, using a horizontal beam.

In addition, the supine anteroposterior projection may produce 'companion shadows', which are superimposed folds of skin and soft-tissue structures that mimic pathological conditions. Often, clinical examination can easily confirm these artefacts created on the radiograph.

## Other views

### Lateral view
The lateral radiograph has a limited role in the investigation of chest trauma. This view is useful for the detection of sternal fractures and for the localization of any foreign bodies. It can be done in a supine patient using the horizontal beam.

### Lateral decubitus

Lateral decubitus examinations of the chest are invaluable in the detection of small pleural or subpulmonic effusions. With the affected side down, free-flowing fluid within the pleural space will become visible along the dependent lateral chest wall. For the detection of pneumothoraces, with the affected side up, the free air should be visible.

### Oblique view

This view is useful for the detection of minimally displaced rib fractures or fractures occurring in the arc of the ribs between the anterior and posterior axillary lines. However, it must be emphasized that radiographs should not be done solely for the detection of rib fractures as the diagnosis of fractures is primarily based on clinical findings. Radiographs, when performed, should be to detect any complications associated with rib fractures.

## Ultrasonography

One of the applications of ultrasound technology is that of two-dimensional echocardiography. This form of investigation is most suitable for the emergency evaluation of cardiac trauma as it is rapid, accurate, non-invasive, and allows for serial examinations. Most importantly, it can be done at the bedside. Clinical uses include the detection of cardiac tamponade, confirmation of electromechanical dissociation (EMD), and diagnosis of haemothorax not apparent on the plain film.

### Cardiac tamponade

The presence of a pericardial effusion after blunt chest injury with a suggestive mechanism should raise the possibility of cardiac tamponade. This is clinically associated with shock, muffled heart sounds, and distended neck veins (Beck's triad).

In the multiple trauma patient with chest injuries, the standard six-view ultrasonography examination allows the detection of cardiac tamponade in the subcostal view. The sonographic detection of pericardial effusion is straightforward and does not require specialized knowledge of echocardiographic cardiac anatomy, standardized cardiac windows, or much experience. The effusion appears as an anechoic space that separates the highly echogenic pericardium from the heart. Findings of a diastolic collapse of the right atrium or ventricle further confirms the presence of tamponade.

Echocardiography often facilitates the performance of pericardiocentesis by guiding the site and direction of needle insertion into the blood-containing pericardial sac.

### EMD confirmation

EMD (electromechanical dissociation) refers to a condition in which an electrical rhythm is present but cardiac wall motion does not occur. The mere absence of a pulse does not mean that true EMD exists. In some instances, the heart may actually be moving but a sufficient pulse pressure is not generated and therefore cannot be palpated clinically. Common causes in trauma include hypovolaemia, tension pneumothorax, and pericardial tamponade. Detection of organized cardiac motion requires only a few seconds and the subcostal view can be used. Findings that refute the diagnosis of EMD are the demonstration of synchronized wall motion or areas of segmental wall motion. Failure to visualize the heart due to intrapleural air suggests the possible diagnosis of tension pneumothorax which may not have been detected clinically.

### Haemothorax

Ultrasonography is not commonly performed to detect haemothorax. The whole process, however, can be completed quickly without moving the patient and haemothorax can be detected by scanning through the lower rib cage. Scanning may be repeated if necessary to assess any bleeding that is not apparent in the initial scan.

In the normal patient, the air-filled lungs prevent much useful information from being obtained. In the presence of an uncomplicated pleural effusion, the appearance is that of an anechoic collection with distal acoustic enhancement which flows freely with any change in the patient's position. Acute haemothorax has the same appearance.

Complicated pleural effusion is seen as fluid collections with septations and perhaps with debris within, and may be loculated. Thickening of the pleural surface may be seen. These features are not unique to haemothorax but are also seen with neoplasms and infection and therefore clinical correlation is essential.

### Transoesophageal echocardiography

This relatively new technique has the advantage of being rapid, minimally invasive, and also allows the visualization of the aortic valve. Its disadvantages include the poor visualization of the distal ascending aorta and interference from the left main-stem bronchus. Special training is required to perform this technique.

## Computed tomography

While conventional radiography is more readily available and provides sufficient information for the majority of chest trauma studies, the CT scan can provide additional information that may aid in subsequent patient management. The benefits of having these details must be weighed against some practical problems, such as the difficulty in monitoring patients during scanning and managing them outside the controlled environment of the emergency department.

Using CT scanning, the diagnostic yield for identification of injuries resulting from trauma to the chest is increased three- to four-fold, compared with plain radiographs alone.

This mode of investigation has the following advantages:

(1)  increased ability to distinguish between soft-tissue structures;

(2)  ability to identify fluid accumulations;

(3)  ability to demonstrate axial relationships;

(4)  ability to delineate individual mediastinal structures;

(5)  diagnosis of pulmonary contusions and diaphragmatic injuries missed in the plain radiographs;

(6)  the course of pulmonary vessels and bronchi can be traced.

In the emergency setting, contrast-enhanced studies are usually not possible, but they allow even greater diagnostic accuracy. The dynamic CT scan with intravenous contrast agents can detect vascular injuries that may not be appreciated on a non-enhanced scan. When the use of oral contrast agents is permissible in a haemodynamically stable, co-operative patient, it increases the yield for diagnosis of oesophageal injuries. In the presence of equivocal findings of mediastinal haematoma on the plain film radiographs, dynamic CT with contrast may be used to demonstrate aortic injury. However, CT findings may be negative in the presence of aortic disruption in some instances, and therefore angiographic studies should be performed in preference when there is a strong clinical suspicion of aortic rupture.

## Angiography

Angiography is the primary imaging modality in the investigation of acute aortic injuries following both penetrating and blunt chest trauma. Surprisingly, such injuries may not result in dramatic physical signs, and may initially be quiescent. Penetrating injuries that do not cause exsanguination can result in false aneurysm formation and arteriovenous (AV) fistulae, and high-energy deceleration injuries may result in aortic tears, where the haematoma is walled in by soft tissues.

Angiography has the advantage of being able to detect subtle injury to the vessel wall and provides information that enables the surgeon to plan and organize appropriate surgical intervention. This modality can be performed safely and quickly. However, angiography allows imaging only of the arterial wall and lumen, and if injuries to other organs are present, they can only be effectively demonstrated using other types of investigation.

To perform angiography, the patient normally has to be moved physically from the emergency department, which may not be safe for an unstable, multiply injured patient. When aortic injury is strongly suspected in a haemodynamically unstable patient, the patient should undergo surgical exploration without this investigation.

## Magnetic resonance imaging

Although deemed one of the most exciting imaging modalities due to the wealth of information it can provide, using MRI for the emergency evaluation of chest trauma is not practical at present. Complete patient co-operation is needed and may be difficult to achieve in the critically ill, and interference with monitoring equipment means that this mode of investigation cannot be performed effectively in this group of patients.

## Other investigations

### Contrast studies

The use of a gastrograffin oesophagram may be useful in the diagnosis of oesophageal injuries in a haemodynamically stable patient. The advantage of gastrograffin over barium sulphate is that it is less irritating if leakage occurs. However, it is known to have a higher false-negative rate in picking up oesophageal perforation.

### Endoscopy

Bronchoscopy is the diagnostic modality of choice for detecting tracheobronchial injuries. Unless the lesions are small, the location and extent of most can be identified. Oesophagoscopy, when performed, is less sensitive than contrast studies in detecting oesophageal perforation.

## IMAGING OF SPECIFIC CONDITIONS

## Chest wall and bony structures

### Clavicular fractures

Isolated clavicular fractures due to blunt trauma are usually quite harmless and diagnosis is straightforward. However, sharp fragments from direct trauma may cause injuries to the subclavian vein, resulting in haematoma or venous thrombosis, and angiography may assist in investigating these complications.

## Rib fractures

Isolated rib fractures occur most frequently from blunt chest trauma. Their frequency increases with age and the amount force required to break the bones decreases as the bones become less elastic.

Injuries usually result from either compression or from a local direct blow to the chest wall. Compression typically produces fractures that buckle outward and injuries to the underlying lung and pleura are infrequent. Direct trauma tends to produce fractures that are inwardly directed and injuries to the underlying structures are more likely.

On the initial radiograph, incomplete or undisplaced fractures may not be identifiable for 7–14 days after injury. Furthermore, injuries to the cartilaginous portions of the ribs may never be seen on radiographs. If the radiological diagnosis of rib fractures is important, oblique views or delayed radiographs may detect fractures not detected initially. It must be emphasized that radiographs should not be performed solely to demonstrate fractures but to detect any associated injuries to the underlying pleural, pulmonary, and visceral structures, or potential complications such as atelectasis and pneumonia.

An upright posteroanterior (P-A) chest radiograph has the highest yield in detecting fractures and associated injuries or complications. Special additional views, such as oblique, coned-down, and tomographic views, should not be performed routinely unless there are specific indications, as in the following situations:

- fractures to ribs 1–3

- fractures to ribs 9–12

- suspicion of multiple rib fractures, especially in the elderly.

Signs of fractures include linear or irregular lucency and cortical disruption or displacement. Unless due to direct trauma, it takes a large amount of force to fracture the first to third ribs, and therefore there may be associated spinal or vascular injuries. Multiple rib fractures are indicators of severe trauma, and the chance of associated intrathoracic trauma increases by about 10 per cent with each rib fractured. The other problem with multiple rib fractures is that of severe pain and the resulting atelectasis and pneumonia from hypoventilation. This is more common in the elderly and in patients with chronic obstructive airway diseases.

When the lower three pairs of ribs are injured, the possibility of intra-abdominal injuries must always be considered.

## Flail chest

A flail chest is present if three or more consecutive ribs are fractured at two or more points. The diagnosis is usually obvious clinically in patients who are adequately exposed. Remember that such injuries can also occur posteriorly and may be missed in a major trauma patient who is supine, unless such injuries are looked for when log rolling the patient. The amount of force necessary to produce a flail segment is very large and hence a search for subtle haemopneumothorax and cardiac and pulmonary contusion is necessary.

## Sternal fractures

Sternal fractures are the result of severe blunt trauma, usually caused by striking the steering wheel in motor vehicle accidents. Sternal fractures are of little signficance by themselves, but due to the amount of force involved, they indicate a significant impact and indicate a great potential for associated serious injuries to the underlying heart or mediastinum. Injuries such as myocardial and pulmonary contusion, vascular disruption, cardiac rupture, and tamponade contribute significantly to the mortality. The type of sternal fracture seen more commonly after the introduction of seat-belt laws tends to have a better prognosis, since it is due to bending forces rather than heavy impact. Clinically, an alert patient would commonly complain of chest pain and findings include bruising and deformity as well as tenderness and crepitus on palpation.

The best view on which to identify these fractures is the lateral chest radiograph (Fig. 12.1). The best clue to the presence of sternal fracture is the presence of a convex soft-tissue mass anterior to the sternum. CT can detect sternal fractures and is also the modality of choice for the evaluation of sternoclavicular dislocations. Multiple cartilaginous or rib fractures adjacent to the sternum can also contribute to the creation of a central flail chest.

Treatment is directed toward management of any coexisting injuries, and because of the association with serious intrathoracic injuries, most patients should be admitted for monitoring after recording a 12-lead electrocardiograph (ECG).

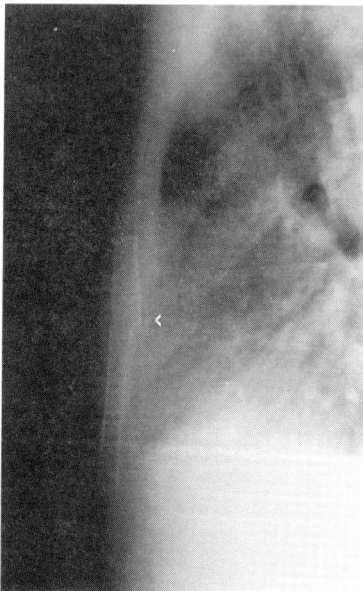

## Injuries to the trachea and major airways

Injuries to the trachea and bronchi may result from either penetrating or blunt forces, and major airway disruption is a rare but potentially fatal complication of chest trauma. Tracheobronchial rupture tends to be unilateral, the incidence of right- and left-sided injuries being equal. About 80 per cent of these injuries occur within 2.5 cm

**Fig. 12.1** Sternum, lateral view: <, sternal fracture with minimal displacement.

either side of the carina, located at the distal trachea or near the origin of a main-stem bronchus.

Increased intrabronchial pressure from an impact to the chest while the glottis is closed may cause rupture of the airway. Other mechanisms include shearing between relatively fixed and mobile structures (between the cricoid cartilage and the carina), traction, and crushing of the airway between an object and vertebral column. Penetrating wounds of the trachea commonly involve the cervical segment and are usually caused by gunshot or stab wounds.

Both clinical and radiological diagnoses of tracheobronchial injury are frequently not recognized and often delayed. Only about one-third of all patients with tracheobronchial disruption are diagnosed in the first 24 hours following injury. The clinical manifestations depend on the location of injury. For example, rupture of the proximal trachea, a very rare injury, may cause haemoptysis and airway obstruction. The presence of symptoms such as shortness of breath, hoarseness of voice, and haemoptysis, together with signs of stridor, cervical emphysema, or pneumothorax, should cause alertness to the possibility of this injury.

On plain radiographs, the signs may be direct or indirect. Direct signs include:

(1)  air may be seen to outline the bronchus;

(2)  the lung may be avulsed from the main-stem bronchus and be seen lying in the dependent portion of the hemithorax (fallen lung sign).

However, most of the plain radiographic evidence of these injuries is indirect, including:

(1)  pneumomediastinum (Fig. 12.2);

(2)  pneumothorax, in some instances tension pneumothorax (Fig. 12.3);

(3)  presence of persistent pneumothorax despite the proper placement of one or more chest tubes;

(4)  subcutaneous emphysema;

(5)  associated injuries such as fractures of the first three ribs, the sternum, and upper thoracic vertebrae.

Up to 10 per cent will have no evidence of bronchial injury on the initial chest radiograph. However, if not treated, almost all of these patients will develop atelectasis within 2–3 weeks as the result of bronchial stenosis. Therefore, delayed radiographs often detect those cases not recognized initially.

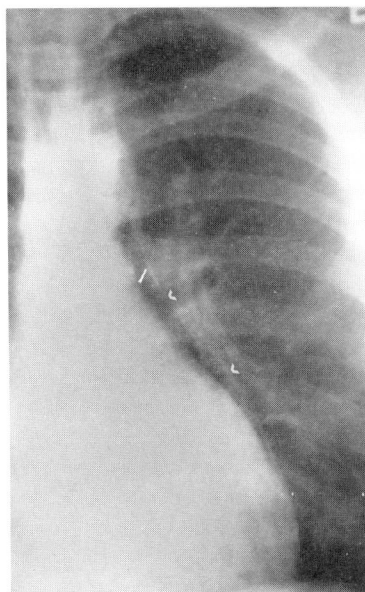

**Fig. 12.2** Chest, frontal view: <, pneumomediastinum.

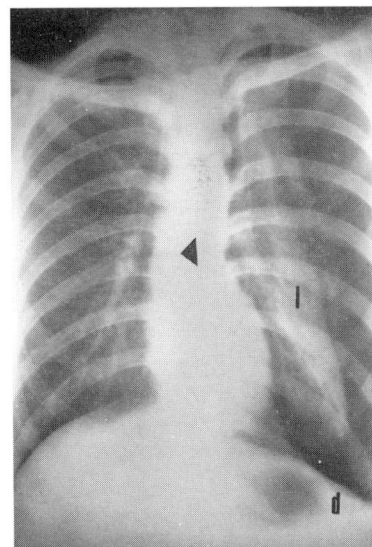

**Fig. 12.3** Chest, frontal view, left tension pneumothorax: ◄, mediastinal shift; l, collapsed lung; d, depressed left hemidiaphragm.

### Other modalities

Fibreoptic bronchoscopy is the diagnostic study of choice for tracheobronchial injury and it is also able to define the extent of the injury. Bronchography is not used in the period of acute injury but may be helpful when the bronchoscopy results are negative and suspicion of injury remains.

A CT scan is helpful for laryngeal injuries but is often not useful for the more distal tracheobronchial injuries.

## Pneumomediastinum

### Causes of pneumomediastinum

1. Pulmonary interstitial emphysema: this is the most common cause of pneumomediastinum in the setting of blunt chest trauma. The alveoli rupture due to a rapid increase in intrathoracic pressure and the air escapes into the interstitial tissue and dissects along interstitial small vessels to enter the mediastinum. This is benign and self-limiting.

2. Tracheobronchial injury: pneumomediastinum occurs frequently in patients with rupture of the major bronchi.

3. Rupture of the oesophagus: this is a rare cause of pneumomediastinum.

### Diagnostic imaging

#### Conventional radiographs
Pneumomediastinum appears as thin, linear, vertically oriented streaks of air outlining mediastinal structures. The left border of the heart is the most common location for the appearance of mediastinal air in adults. The aortic knob, the great vessels, the aortic pulmonic window, and descending aorta may be outlined by the free air. The central portion of the diaphragm, usually obscured by the heart, may sometimes be outlined by the air, producing the continuous diaphragm sign.

Air may extend from the mediastinum into the peritoneal cavity or into the retroperitoneum. It can also dissect superiorly along the fascial planes into the neck. Most commonly, such deep cervical emphysema is seen anterior to the prevertebral fascia and appears as a linear stripe of air just anterior to the cervical spine.

If pneumomediastinum is suspected on a chest film, a lateral view of the cervical spine may produce convincing, confirmatory proof.

# Injuries to the lung parenchyma and pleura

## Pulmonary contusion

Pulmonary contusion usually occurs as a result of blunt chest wall trauma. It occurs typically in deceleration injury from motor vehicle accidents and is associated with falls and non-penetrating missile and concussive injuries. In the presence of rib or sternal fractures, the possibility of pulmonary contusion must be considered, although it can occur without any associated bony involvement. When a flail chest is found, it should be assumed that pulmonary contusion is always present.

Pathologically, the contusion is characterized by interstitial oedema with capillary damage and intra-alveolar extravasation of protein and blood from the ruptured microvessels. These collections may be large enough to produce patchy alveolar infiltrates on the chest radiograph. Increased secretions result in atelectasis and consolidation, which prevent the rapid resolution of these changes. The basic structural integrity of the lung is maintained in simple contusion.

### *Diagnostic imaging*

The major disadvantage of relying on the initial chest radiograph is that changes lag behind the patient's physiological condition and the diagnosis of pulmonary contusion may be missed in some patients. The infiltrate of pulmonary contusion is usually present within 6 hours of the time of injury and may often not be seen on the first chest X-ray obtained in the A&E department.

On the radiographs, the opaque infiltrates may either be discrete or confluent and differ from the those seen after aspiration by their lack of anatomical confinement to particular lobes or segments. The infiltrates may be very extensive, may be bilateral, and even be suggestive of a contracoup mechanism location. The opacification may worsen for up to 48 hours (usually the first 24 hours) after the initial injury and most contusions begin to clear radiographically within 72 hours. Persistent progression of shadowing after this period is often due to superimposed problems such as atelectasis, pneumonia, and pulmonary infarction.

In the presence of developing clinical signs of contusion, such as progressive hypoxia, increasing respiratory rate, and carbon dioxide retention, in the absence of radiological signs on the chest film, a CT scan of the chest should be considered. CT scanning is the most sensitive imaging modality for diagnosis of pulmonary contusion, allowing the clinician to detect areas of contusion before they become evident on plain chest films.

## Pulmonary laceration and haematoma

Pulmonary lacerations in blunt trauma result from shearing forces that disrupt the lung parenchyma and vessels. A large amount of force is required to produce these injuries. When the lacerations are filled with blood, they result in pulmonary haematomas. In a similar way, a pneumatocoele may result when the spaces are filled with air. Often both fluid and air are present in the spaces.

Radiologically, these areas may be completely obscured by surrounding lung contusion, and become evident only as the contusion clears. They appear initially as fuzzy, indistinct lesions that progress to distinct nodules over days before resolving, usually without sequelae. They vary in size from one to several centimetres. The changes may be widespread and bilateral as parenchymal damage does not respect lobar boundaries. Appropriately, the changes may be most severe adjacent to the regions of skeletal damage, or under the point of impact. Small haematomas and lacerations may be missed on the chest film.

## Pneumothorax

Pneumothorax is typically categorized as simple, open, or tension. A simple pneumothorax is one that neither connects with the external chest nor demonstrates a progressive accumulation of air in the pleural space.

A pneumothorax is not prone to cause severe symptoms in an otherwise healthy patient unless it develops tension and occupies more than 40 per cent of one hemithorax, but it may, however, manifest early in patients with shock or pre-existing cardiopulmonary disease. If there is a suspicion of a pneumothorax, but it is not clearly seen on the first chest radiograph, repeat films during expiration may be helpful. Very occasionally a delayed pneumothorax may occur 12–24 hours after a penetrating wound, and late presentations after several weeks, usually following exertion, have occurred.

Pneumothorax occurs as a result of blunt trauma in 15–50 per cent of patients. It occurs most commonly from pleural violation by associated rib fractures, but may also result from a ruptured bleb, alveolus, or bronchus. Penetrating trauma may introduce air through the wound track or through a lung-tissue laceration.

When the chest radiograph is taken in the upright position, the radiographic diagnosis is usually made based on the appearance of a thin pleural line in the apex and the apicolateral aspect of the lung with absence of lung markings beyond the pleural line. When the chest film is taken during expiration, it often enhances a small pneumothorax, owing both to the positive pressure and the smaller volume of the lung. Decubitus radiographs with the suspected side up are sometimes useful in confirming the presence of a small pneumothorax.

In severely injured patients, the chest radiographs can only be obtained in the supine position and the recognition of pneumothorax is more difficult. The radiograph taken may not show the classic appearance of an apicolateral air collection. In this position, air collects in the highest portion of the chest, which is the anterior costophrenic sulcus.

The signs in this view include:

(1) hyperlucency of the upper abdominal quadrants and lower chest;

(2) a deep costophrenic sulcus appearance;

(3) double diaphragm contour;

(4) presence of a sharply defined pericardial fat pad and a distinct cardiac apex;

(5) subpulmonic location of air which outlines the visceral pleura of the lung base.

When interpreting radiographs it is wise to be aware of the possible artefacts that mimic pneumothorax; for example, skin folds that simulate pleural lines. Skin folds produce an edge of radiodensity, often with a thin black line seen just to the outside, which is unlike the very thin, sharp line produced by the displaced visceral pleura of a pneumothorax. When the line is produced by a skin fold, lung markings extend beyond its edge. The edges produced by skin folds often start and stop abruptly as the skin fold merges with the adjacent chest surface. Skin folds are often multiple, and they may extend across the midline or outside the rib cage. In cases of doubt, a repeat chest film is helpful as skin folds generally disappear or change location considerably with differences in patient positioning. Other artefacts include pleural blebs and superimposed clothing and debris on the trolley.

## Tension pneumothorax

This is a pneumothorax that is under pressure, causing a shift in the mediastinal structures away from the affected side, with gradual reduction in venous return to the heart. If left untreated, this can progress rapidly to decreased cardiac output, haemodynamic collapse, and eventual death. It must be emphasized that in the presence of clinical signs (decreased breath sounds, respiratory distress, hypotension, and tachycardia), treatment should be given *before* the taking of the chest radiographs. However, as the pressure around the collapsed lung takes time to rise, a chest radiograph may reveal the shift in mediastinal structures before the patient begins to show any clinical signs of a tension pneumothorax. The size of a pneumothorax is not a reliable indicator of tension on its own. In patients undergoing mechanical ventilation, tension may develop rapidly and with a smaller appearance on the radiograph.

Radiographic signs of tension include contralateral displacement of mediastinal structures, depression of the ipsilateral hemidiaphragm, hyperinflated hemithorax, and atelectasis of adjacent lung tissue.

### Haemothorax

Haemothorax results from bleeding into the pleural space from rupture of blood vessels in the chest wall, the pleura, the lung, the mediastinum, or the diaphragm. Haemothorax caused by bleeding from small vessels tends to be moderate in size. A fast-expanding haemothorax is usually due to a major systemic or pulmonary artery injury. Major haemorrhage from laceration of the lung following blunt trauma is usually caused by the sharp ends of fractured ribs.

The radiographic findings include:

1. Diffuse unilateral haziness. This is the result of the blood and fluid collecting posteriorly. No air bronchogram effect is present and vascular markings can frequently be seen through the pleural fluid. This differs from the signs of parenchymal disease, which obliterate normal vascular markings and often produce air bronchograms.

2. Thickened pleura or a widened paraspinal stripe. The dependent fluid can appear indirectly as thickened pleura, and the widening of the paraspinous stripe is caused by fluid layering medially in a supine patient.

3. It is important to note that up to 1000 ml of blood may collect before haemothorax becomes apparent on the supine radiograph.

When the radiograph is taken in a upright position, a fluid collection of greater than 250 ml can usually be seen on good-quality films. This will appear as blunting of the costophrenic angle, and the diaphragm is often obscured by the adjacent fluid. Fluid may extend over the apex of the lung to produce an apical pleural cap. As the amount of free fluid in the chest increases, the ipsilateral lung undergoes progressive parenchymal compression and atelectasis. Sometimes, penetrating injuries may result in haemopneumothorax, which is indicated by a horizontal line in the erect chest radiograph and indicates the need for urgent decompression by tube thoracostomy.

The decubitus view is useful in confirming the presence and the size of pleural fluid collections. It allows the detection of haemothorax in a patient who is too ill to be placed in the erect position.

# Injuries to heart

Penetrating injuries of the heart may be rapidly fatal but small wounds may self-seal or bleed slowly. The presence of a penetrating chest wound between the mid-clavicular line on the right and the mid-axillary line on the left should raise the possibility of a cardiac injury.

Radiology plays only a minor role in the diagnosis of penetrating injuries to the heart. Very rarely, a chest radiograph may show intrapericardial air. Often it is performed simply to record the presence and location of the penetrating object, such as an impaling stake or knife blade. Other associated injuries may be diagnosed, for example the presence of haemopneumothorax.

## Myocardial rupture and acute cardiac tamponade

Myocardial rupture is rare and survivors are few. Of those who survive to reach the Accident and Emergency department, the mechanism is usually chest impact in a motor vehicle accident. On rare occasions it may occur suddenly and unpredictably about 2 weeks after myocardial contusion, when myonecrosis leads to softening and rupture.

Acute cardiac tamponade should be suspected in any patient who presents with a penetrating wound to the chest or upper abdomen and demonstrates signs of an elevated central venous pressure, shock, and tachycardia after tension pneumothorax has been excluded.

A history of chest pain followed by rapid deterioration may be present, but other injuries may mask the picture. If the pericardium remains intact, the patient will present with signs of cardiac tamponade. If the pericardium ruptures together with the heart, the patient would normally not survive to reach hospital. An exception might be a limited penetrating wound which opens both the pericardium and heart, which may cause free bleeding and signs of shock without tamponade.

If the diagnosis of myocardial rupture is suspected, most diagnostic studies are superfluous and the only definitive treatment is operative repair. Pericardiocentesis may be attempted as a temporizing measure in the patient who has vital signs, but a negative procedure does not exclude tamponade. If the patient loses vital signs, immediate emergency department thoracotomy is indicated.

### Radiological examination

Plain chest radiography is not useful in the diagnosis of myocardial rupture and cardiac tamponade. The cardiac shadow is usually normal even in the presence of acute tamponade.

Echocardiography is a non-invasive bedside study which can be used to detect pericardial fluid and is useful for a patient who is haemodynamically unstable. Again, however, investigation should not delay the treatment in a patient suspected of myocardial rupture.

CT is useful in those patients who have remained stable following a penetrating injury but where the wounding mechanism suggests a high risk of heart or mediastinal involvement, as with stab wounds and gunshot injuries.

## Myocardial contusion

Cardiac contusion results from blunt trauma and ranges from mild surface contusion to severe transmural contusion. Clinically, it may result in myocardial dysfunction which produces low cardiac output and a risk of acute cardiac arrhythmia. With the more severe injuries, congestive failure or cardiac rupture may occur. Although cardiac contusion is common in those patients sustaining blunt anterior chest trauma, most of these patients only exhibit electrocardiographic abnormalities and raised cardiac enzyme levels, with no increase in mortality. Often the cardiac abnormalities are missed or the diagnosis delayed as they are masked by more obvious injuries. Coronary arteries can also be injured directly after blunt chest trauma, leading to spasm, pseudoaneurysm formation, intimal injury, or occlusion.

The presence of anterior rib fractures and sternal fractures should raise suspicion of myocardial injury, although there is no clear relationship between the extent of chest wall injury and the degree of underlying cardiac damage. The right ventricle is most commonly affected and may develop transient segmental wall abnormalities.

It should be suspected when the following clinical features are present:

(1)  any patient involved in a motor vehicle accident at speeds exceeding 35 mph and in the presence of any chest symptoms or signs of significant chest wall injury;

(2)  a tachycardia that is out of proportion to the degree of trauma or blood loss;

(3)  a patient having angina-like pain that is not relieved by nitroglycerine;

(4)  the presence of other physical signs such as a friction rub or abnormality in the heart sounds;

(5)  the presence of an acute arrhythmia such as atrial fibrillation or multiple premature atrial or ventricular contractions.

### *Diagnostic imaging*

The main problem with myocardial contusion is that there is no 'standard' modality to establish the diagnosis. The following are some of the modalities used.

*Conventional radiography* The value of chest radiograph lies only in the recognition of associated injuries that might raise the suspicion of myocardial contusion. The closest radiographic correlations are pulmonary contusion or fractures of the first two ribs, the clavicles, or the sternum. The presence of a fractured sternum due to impact is the most significant. The presence of acute pulmonary oedema associated with a normal-sized heart should raise the suspicion of acute cardiac decompensation. The cardiac silhouette is usually not enlarged in cardiac tamponade but a widened azygos vein is suggestive of this diagnosis.

*Technetium-99 scans* Radionuclide scanning using the technetium-labelled pyrophosphate is based on the principle that the isotope binds to damaged cardiac cells and can identify contused myocardium. However, it lacks sensitivity as a transmural injury is necessary to make the study interpretable, since enough scintigraphic tracer needs to be bound in order to distinguish the lesion from background noise. It is further limited by obscuring structures, such as the overlying sternum or chest-wall contusions.

*SPECT* Single photon emission computed tomography (SPECT) displays computerized thallium chloride ($^{201}$TlCl$_3$) images of the heart, taken as tomographic slides in different planes. Compared to conventional $^{201}$TlCl$_3$ imaging, this modality greatly increases the diagnostic accuracy.

*Radionuclide angiography* Radionuclide angiography uses a first-pass examination of left or right ventricular ejections and segmental wall motion to demonstrate myocardial function dynamically. This technique is rapid, non-invasive, can be performed at the bedside, and appears to be both sensitive and specific in making the diagnosis. Its disadvantage is that it needs sophisticated equipment and is therefore expensive and often not readily available.

*Echocardiography* Two-dimensional echocardiography provides rapid, accurate, non-invasive, and relatively inexpensive diagnostic information, both quantitatively and qualitatively. Information can be gained on the status of the cardiac chambers, wall motion abnormalities, functional integrity of the valves, and the presence of cardiac tamponade and intracardiac thrombus or shunts. It can differentiate between right and left ventricular contusions. The most common abnormality seen with myocardial contusion is right ventricular free-wall dyskinesia, usually with some dilation of the chamber. Technical limitations due to movement and surgical dressings may lead to inadequate studies in some patients.

**Traumatic rupture of the aorta**

Thoracic vascular trauma may result from rapid deceleration in motor vehicle accidents, a fall from height, or from a direct penetrating wound. The most common site of aortic injury is at the proximal descending aorta, just distal to the left subclavian artery and in the region of the ligamentum arteriosum. The majority of patients with acute aortic injury sustain free rupture of the full thickness of the aorta. These patients exsanguinate at the moment of injury and consequently they rarely present as a clinical or radiological emergency. In patients who survive this injury, the aorta is not completely ruptured but its wall is torn, with the adventitial layer still preserving the integrity of the aorta for a period of time. The rupture of the resultant aneurysm may occur at any time, from within the first 24 hours of injury to a few weeks after. Early diagnosis is therefore vital to prevent rupture before surgical repair can be carried out.

*Diagnostic imaging*

*Conventional radiography*  The most sensitive radiographic sign of traumatic thoracic aortic rupture on the routine anteroposterior chest film is a widened mediastinum of more than 8 cm above the level of the carina, which is seen in over 90 per cent of patients. Alternatively, a mediastinum that extends for more than 25 per cent of the width of the chest at this level can be presumed abnormal. However, the specificity of this sign is low and other radiological signs indicating mediastinal haemorrhage and possible aortic rupture should be sought. These include:

(1)  blurring of the aortic knob;

(2)  opacification of the aortopulmonary space;

(3)  tracheal deviation;

(4)  the presence of fluid in the left pleural space;

(5)  a left apical pleural cap;

(6)  depression of the left main-stem bronchus;

(7)  deviation of the nasogastric tube shadow to the right;

(8)  widening of the right paratracheal stripe and the paraspinal lines.

Unfortunately, none of the signs has significant sensitivity or specificity to preclude the need to use angiography. In a proportion of patients, a widened mediastinum and other radiological changes may not be apparent on the chest X-ray for several hours.

The optimal chest radiograph is an upright P-A film taken at 6 feet

(1.83 m) with good inspiration. This is usually not possible in patients who sustain major trauma. A false appearance of mediastinal widening may be seen if the radiograph is obtained anteroposteriorly, less than 100 cm from the X-ray machine, with the patient lying supine and with poor inspiration.

*CT and angiography*   Thoracic aortography is the most sensitive investigation and is the gold standard for defining the site of disruption. However, it will not delineate the size of a mediastinal haematoma or define the site of venous bleeding. The preselection criteria should be based on the findings of non-invasive studies, such as plain chest radiography or CT. While a CT scan is very sensitive for detecting the presence of mediastinal haemorrhage, it has poor specificity and must be followed immediately by angiography in order to determine the presence and location of any aortic or great vessel injury. Few cardiothoracic surgeons are prepared to operate without an aortogram, and the longer the delay, the greater will be the chance of the patient succumbing to the injury. If aortic disruption is highly suspected on the plain radiographs, the aortogram and surgical intervention should take precedence over other imaging and treatment of other injuries that are not immediately life threatening.

The high percentage of normal angiograms in the investigation of possible aortic disruption is to be expected as there is a tendency to obtain aortograms even when there is only a slight suspicion of aortic disruption. This does not reflect badly on the judgement of the physician since no clinical or plain radiographic features can reliably substitute for the investigation.

## Injury to the oesophagus

Oesophageal injury caused by external trauma is relatively uncommon except in the cervical segment, and injuries caused by penetrating mechanisms are the most common at this site. Whether caused by blunt or penetrating trauma, oesophageal injury is rarely isolated, and the trachea is the most common associated site involved. Associated injuries may have a more dramatic presentation and therefore the oesophageal injury may be overlooked initially. Delayed treatment of oesophageal injury is associated with prolonged morbidity and increased mortality rates.

Oesophageal rupture following blunt trauma seems to be caused by the violent ejection of stomach contents in the presence of a tightly closed cricopharyngeus muscle acting as a sphincter. Perforation is usually the result of instrumentation or swallowed foreign bodies. The initial symptoms of oesophageal rupture are subtle and non-specific and may be missed easily in patients sustaining multiple trauma.

Most commonly, patients have substernal pleuritic pain radiating to the neck or shoulders and there may be shortness of breath and dysphagia. Early signs include pneumothorax, rhythmic Hamman's sign and subcutaneous emphysema. If undiagnosed, fever and mediastinitis may set in, due to the inflammation associated with the contaminated spillage. Perforations of the oesophagus have been referred to as the most rapidly fatal perforation of the gastrointestinal tract.

The mortality is dependent on several variables: mechanism of injury, location of the oesophageal perforation, the time elapsed between injury and diagnosis, presence of pre-existing oesophageal disease, and the general health of the patient.

### Conventional radiography

Lateral views of the cervical spine are helpful in detecting blood or air in the retropharyngeal space. Perforations in the lower parts of the oesophagus may release fluid that dissects superiorly into the neck, so the radiological signs may not help in localizing the site of injury.

The chest radiographs of patients who have an oesophageal rupture may be normal initially but clues to the diagnosis may be present on careful inspection of the film. These include:

(1)   pneumomediastinum   with   or   without   subcutaneous emphysema;

(2)   left-sided pleural effusion;

(3)   pneumothorax or hydropneumothorax;

(4)   widened mediastinum.

### Contrast studies and endoscopy

Gastrograffin oesophagram is the preferred initial contrast study. Gastrograffin will not affect visualization if endoscopy is performed later and it produces less mediastinal damage than barium if leakage occurs.

Endoscopy is a less sensitive study and results very much depend on the expertise of the operator and the availability. Some authors recommend endoscopy initially, to be followed by a gastrograffin oesophagram if endoscopy is negative.

## Diaphragmatic rupture

Most diaphragmatic injuries result from direct penetration of the diaphragm. Blunt diaphragmatic rupture generally results from severe trauma, and mortality rates in patients with this condition are around 20–25 per cent.

Diaphragmatic injuries may not be clinically obvious until much later. It is usually the herniation of abdominal contents into the chest, leading to complications of visceral incarceration, obstruction, ischaemia from strangulation, or perforation that makes the diagnosis obvious. The delay in diagnosis may result in some cases from confounding radiological signs, such as lung contusion, pneumatocoele, and pleural fluid.

Following blunt trauma, rupture of the diaphragm usually occurs at the domes and is more common on the left, as the liver acts as a cushion on the right. The tears resulting from blunt trauma are larger than those of penetrating injury. Stab wounds of the diaphragm are also more often on the left (presumably due to a predominance of right-handed assailants) although gunshot wounds are more evenly distributed between the sides.

The clinical presentation of diaphragmatic rupture progresses through three phrases: early, latent, and late phase. In the early phase, symptoms include chest pain radiating to the left shoulder, shortness of breath, and abdominal pain, and signs include scaphoid abdomen, bowel sounds in the chest, ipsilateral diminished breath sounds, inability to pass a nasogastric tube into the stomach, and failure to recover lavage effluent when diagnostic peritoneal lavage is performed. The latent phase occurs when the diagnosis is not made during the initial presentation and typically the patient has vague intermittent abdominal pain; this would progress to the late phase if the diagnosis is again not made. By then, obstruction or strangulation of the herniated contents may occur.

## Conventional radiography and contrast studies

The chest radiograph is the most useful initial study and it is usually performed routinely in a multiply injured patient as part of a trauma series. However, diagnostic signs are present in only half of the patients with diaphragmatic injuries, and any abnormality of the diaphragm or left lower lung field in the setting of blunt trauma should arouse the suspicion of a tear. The chest films may demonstrate bowel gas or loops of intestine above the diaphragm, or if a nasogastric tube is inserted, the presence of its tip above the diaphragm. The hemidiaphragm may be obscured or elevated as the herniated intestine flattens under the lung. The mediastinum may be shifted. Associated fractures of the lower ribs and pneumothorax, haemothorax, or atelectasis may be seen. If the initial chest radiograph is negative, subsequent films may be needed as the visceral herniation may be intermittent.

The presence of a contrast-filled viscus above the diaphragm in a barium contrast study, or bowel obstruction at the level of the diaphragm, is diagnostic.

### Ultrasonography and CT

Both the CT scan and ultrasound have been used to diagnose acute diaphragmatic injuries, but sensitivity is poor for injuries without herniation of abdominal contents. On ultrasonographic examinations, the diaphragm is a readily identifiable structure and the herniated bowel can be identified by its peristaltic activity. The herniation of solid abdominal contents, such as liver or omentum, can also be identified.

CT scanning cannot identify the actual rupture but can identify herniation through it. Often CT is performed in the investigation of abdominal and pelvic trauma, and isolated cases of diaphragmatic herniation are identified incidentally.

The other problems associated with the use of CT and ultrasound result from distension of the herniated stomach, which is either due to a partial volvulus or post-traumatic acute dilatation. The interface of the stomach with lung may resemble a normal but markedly elevated diaphragm, and thus the true diagnosis may be missed. However, the insertion of a nasogastric tube will indicate the herniation.

### MRI

Magnetic resonance imaging allows for good visualization of the diaphragm. However, the lack of easy availability and interference with monitoring devices make this suitable only in haemodynamically stable patients.

## Chest trauma in children—points to note

The most common mechanism of chest injuries in children is blunt trauma and is usually associated with motor vehicle accidents. The incidence of penetrating chest injuries is low.

Due to the increased elasticity and compliance of the chest wall, the incidence of rib fractures, sternal fractures, and flail chest in children is much lower. This increased chest wall compliance also means that traumatic forces are transmitted to the underlying organs with little or no sign of chest-wall trauma, and significant pulmonary and myocardial contusions may occur in the absence of rib fractures. As a corollary, where rib fractures are found in children, the amount of force must necessarily have been significant and the associated risk of severe underlying injuries is increased.

In children, the presence of a stable pneumothorax of 15 per cent or less, which is asymptomatic, may be treated conservatively by close observation, as the majority of pneumothoraces of this size resorb spontaneously. However, pneumothorax in a child is more prone to progress to a tension pneumothorax, due to the increased mobility of the mediastinal structures, and close observation is necessary.

## Summary

Algorithms for the evaluation of chest injuries and suspected aortic disruption are given in Figs 12.4 and 12.5, respectively.

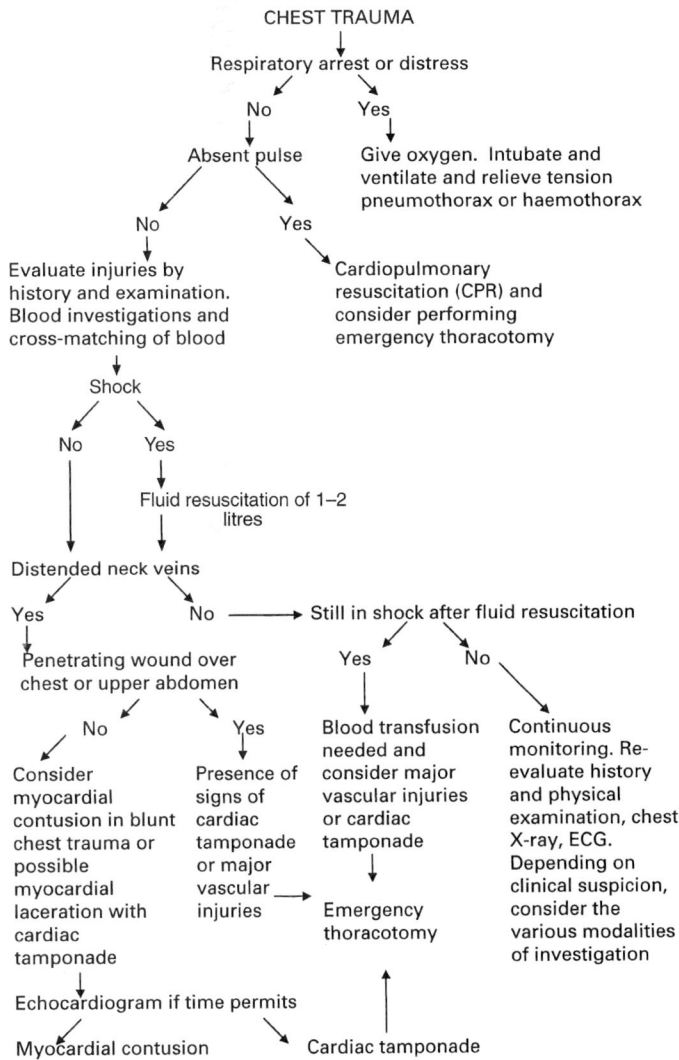

CHEST TRAUMA

Respiratory arrest or distress

No — Yes

Absent pulse — Give oxygen. Intubate and ventilate and relieve tension pneumothorax or haemothorax

No — Yes

Evaluate injuries by history and examination. Blood investigations and cross-matching of blood — Cardiopulmonary resuscitation (CPR) and consider performing emergency thoracotomy

Shock

No — Yes

Fluid resuscitation of 1–2 litres

Distended neck veins

Yes — No ⟶ Still in shock after fluid resuscitation

Yes — No

Penetrating wound over chest or upper abdomen

No — Yes | Blood transfusion needed and consider major vascular injuries or cardiac tamponade | Continuous monitoring. Re-evaluate history and physical examination, chest X-ray, ECG. Depending on clinical suspicion, consider the various modalities of investigation

Consider myocardial contusion in blunt chest trauma or possible myocardial laceration with cardiac tamponade | Presence of signs of cardiac tamponade or major vascular injuries | Emergency thoracotomy

Echocardiogram if time permits

Myocardial contusion — Cardiac tamponade

**Fig. 12.4** Algorithm for the evaluation of chest injuries.

Aortic disruption suspected from mechanism of injury

Chest radiograph

Normal          Equivocal          Abnormal

Observe     A repeat film and P-A     Angiography
            erect if possible

        Normal     Equivocal     Abnormal

            Observe     Mechanism is highly
                        suspicious

                    No          Yes

                CT scan     Angiography

            Normal     Abnormal

                    Angiography

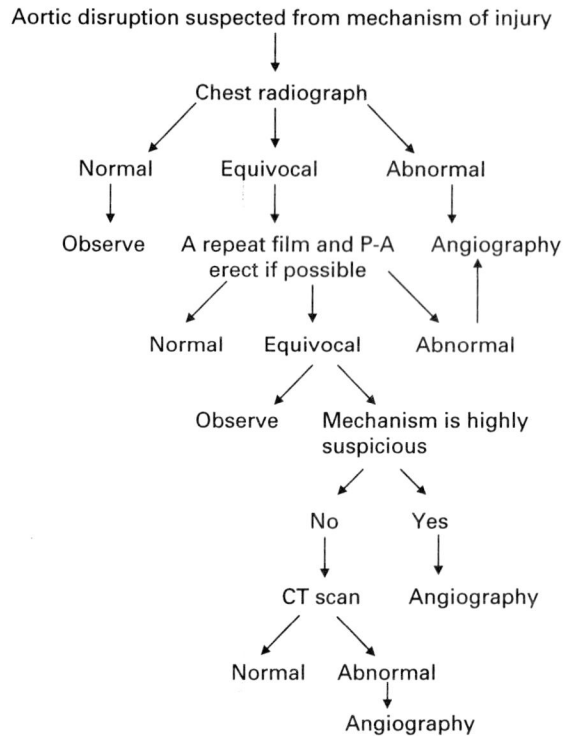

**Fig. 12.5**   Algorithm for the evaluation of suspected aortic disruption.

# BIBLIOGRAPHY

Ballinger PW. Merrill's Atlas of Radiographic Positions and Radiologic Procedures, 8th edn. Missouri: Mosby, 1995; 1: 399–480.

Ballinger PW, Rutherford RB, Zuidema GD. The Management of Trauma. Philadelphia: WB Saunders, 1968.

Charkravarty M. Utilisation of aortography in trauma. Radiol Clin North Am 1986; 24(3):383–96.

Ellis, H. Clinical Anatomy, 8th edn. Oxford: Blackwell Scientific Publications, 1992.

Goodman PC. CT of chest trauma. In: Federle MP, Brandt-Zawadski M, eds. Computed Tomography in the Evaluation of Trauma, 2nd edm. Baltimore: Williams & Wilkins, 1986.

Grumback K, Mechlin M, Mintz M. Computed tomography and ultrasound of the traumatised and acutely ill patient. Emerg Med Clin North Am 1985; 3(3):607–24.

Heitzman ER. The Mediastinum: Radiologic Correlation with Anatomy and Pathology, 2nd edn. Berlin: Springer-Velag, 1988.

Henry DA. Thoracic trauma: radiologic triage of the chest radiography. Am Roentgen Ray Soc 1987; April:13–22.

Hood RM, Boyd AD, Culliford AT. Thoracic Trauma. Philadelphia: WB Saunders, 1989.

Lundervall J. The mechanism of traumatic rupture of the aorta. Acta Pathol Microbiol Scand 1964; 62:34–46.

Marnocha KE, Maglinte DDT. Plain film criteria for excluding aortic rupture in blunt chest trauma. AJR 1985; 144:19–21.

Meschan IA. An Atlas of Anatomy Basic to Radiology. Philadelphia: WB Saunders, 1975.

Mirvis SE. Imaging of thoracic trauma. In: Yurney SZ, Rodriguez A, Cowley RA, eds. Management of Cardiothoracic Trauma. Baltimore: Williams & Wilkins, 1990.

Sefczek DM, Sefczek RJ, Deeb ZL. Radiographic signs of acute traumatic rupture of the thoracic aorta. AJR 1983; 141:1259–62.

Sivit CJ, Taylor GA, Eichelberger MR. Chest injury in children with blunt abdominal trauma: evaluation with CT. Radiology 1989; 171:815–18.

Van Moor A, Ravin CE, Putman CE. Radiologic evaluation of acute chest trauma. CRC Crit Rev Diagn Imaging 1983; 19:89–110.

# CHAPTER 13

# *The abdomen*

- Key points: the abdomen
- Clinical anatomy
- Clinical assessment
- The techniques available
- Imaging of specific injuries
- Bibliography

---

## Key points: the abdomen

1. Supine radiographs of the abdomen are not performed routinely as part of the initial radiograph series, and are of little value in blunt trauma. They may be useful in locating fragmented missiles or retained bullets caused by gunshot injuries or other projectiles.

2. If erect examination is not possible, a decubitus film with the right side up may show free air accumulation along the right lobe of the liver.

3. Ultrasonography is being used increasingly in the investigation of abdominal trauma. It is non-invasive, portable, and can be repeated whenever necessary. It is especially useful in patients who are haemodynamically unstable and cannot be transferred to the CT suite.

4. Six-view ultrasound examinations are valuable for detection of haemoperitoneum and cardiac tamponade in multiple trauma patients.

5. CT provides anatomical views of the entire abdomen, including the pelvic structures and retroperitoneum, with excellent resolution, and is useful in evaluating abdominal trauma. It is probably the best examination available, but the logistics of moving the patient may create hazards. Basing a CT scanner in the A&E department increases its usefulness.

*(Continued)*

6. Magnetic resonance imaging is not suitable for the initial evaluation of abdominal injuries and is restricted to stable patients who do not need continuous life-support monitoring devices.

7. In genitourinary injuries, radiological examination is often needed for definitive diagnosis. Certain physical signs such as contusions or abrasions over the flanks or lower abdomen, lower rib fracture, perineal swelling, or scrotal haematoma should raise the suspicion of renal or urinary-tract injuries. Haematuria by itself has poor correlation with the injury severity.

8. A bedside 7-minute intravenous pyelogram (IVP) can be performed for assessment of urinary-tract injuries when computed tomography (CT) is not available or the patient is too unstable for CT.

9. Bladder injuries often occur in association with pelvic fractures, due to their close anatomical relationship, and occur more frequently when the bladder is full at the time of the accident.

## CLINICAL ANATOMY

Anatomically, the abdomen is the portion of the body that lies below the diaphragm and above the pelvic inlet. By using abdominal lines and planes, the abdomen is divided into nine regions. In the upper abdomen are the right hypochondrium, epigastrium, and left hypochondrium. In the middle abdomen, the right lumbar, umbilical, and left lumbar regions are located. In the lower abdomen, the right iliac region, hypogastrium, and left iliac regions are located. The significance of this division is that in each of these regions specific organs are located, and thus potential injuries can be classified and better described. The liver lies in the right hypochondrium above the costal margin. The level of its upper border varies with respiration, and may reach the fourth intercostal space on expiration. Its left lobe passes below the xiphisternum across the epigastrium. The spleen is in the left hypochondrium, situated posterolaterally along the line of the left ninth to eleventh ribs.

The peritoneum is a thin, serous membrane lining the walls and organs of the abdomen and pelvis. The parietal peritoneum lines the walls of the abdominal and pelvic cavities, and visceral peritoneum covers the organs. The potential space between the parietal and visceral layers of peritoneum is termed the peritoneal cavity. Retroperitoneal organs are those lying behind the peritoneal cavity or covered only in the front by peritoneum. Examples of these include the pancreas, duodenum, ascending and descending colon, the inferior vena cava, and the aorta. Some injuries to these retroperitoneal organs may not be detected easily because there is no bleeding into the peritoneal cavity to cause irritation and physical signs.

The peritoneal cavity is divided into an upper part within the abdomen and a lower part in the pelvis. The abdominal part is further subdivided by the many peritoneal reflections into fossae and spaces, such as the subphrenic and subhepatic spaces. When haemorrhage occurs from injured organs, blood collects in these spaces.

The kidneys are paired, bean-shaped organs that are retroperitoneal and lie on each side of the vertebral column in the upper abdomen. The left kidney is usually higher than the right and, in the majority of people, the right kidney is slightly smaller than the left.

There is considerable mobility of the kidneys during respiration. The range of movement is larger for women than for men. On deep inspiration excursions of up to 10 cm have been recorded.

The ureter connects the kidney to the bladder and is also a retroperitoneal structure. It measures about 25 cm in length, has a fairly constant course and slight anatomical constrictions at the following sites:

- pelvic–ureteric junction in the kidney
- where the ureter crosses the pelvic brim
- the intramural portion in the bladder.

The urinary bladder lies posterior to the pubic symphysis, which makes it vulnerable to injury when the symphysis or pubic rami are fractured.

The female urethra is short when compared to that of the male and as such it is seldom injured by trauma to the pelvis. The male urethra is longer and is divided into prostatic, membranous, and cavernous portions.

## CLINICAL ASSESSMENT

The main purpose of an abdominal examination in the early phase after trauma is to identify the presence of any signs of injuries requiring early surgical management, and the precise diagnosis of specific injuries is only of secondary importance. In some cases, physical findings are unreliable due to head injury, intoxication, or spinal-cord injury.

The diagnosis of intra-abdominal injury must be placed within a systematic and orderly evaluation and resuscitation of the patient. Other significant injuries, for example to the airway, chest, heart, or great vessels may also occur, and these injuries may take precedence in terms of diagnosis and management.

A careful management plan is needed to prioritize investigations and treatment, as the timely use of diagnostic procedures and vigorous therapy directed at life-threatening conditions will positively influence both mortality and morbidity. Resuscitation and stabilization must always precede any radiological investigations. A seriously injured patient who requires radiographic investigations in the radiology department should be accompanied by trained personnel and should not be left unmonitored even for a brief period. Often, for haemodynamically unstable patients with abdominal injuries, laparotomy should be performed rather than imaging studies.

## Blunt and penetrating trauma

Blunt trauma tends to carry a higher mortality than penetrating injury for a variety of reasons. Diagnosis is often more difficult in blunt trauma and it is commonly associated with severe trauma to other organ systems. Other more obvious signs in these systems may mask the seemingly trivial features of abdominal injuries in the early phase after trauma.

In blunt trauma, solid-organ injury may be due to direct compressive force, from sudden deceleration which may avulse vascular and mesenteric attachments, or to laceration by bony fragments from adjacent fractures. Sudden compressive force may also result in injury to hollow viscera by increasing the intraluminal pressure, causing the intestinal wall to burst or blood vessels to be disrupted.

Although the accuracy of physical examination is limited in many cases, it still has an important place in assessing abdominal trauma, especially in a fully conscious, haemodynamically stable patient. Certain injuries that may cause few symptoms initially, for example bowel perforations and pancreatic contusions, become progressively symptomatic within a short period and may be detected by serial abdominal examinations. However, retroperitoneal injuries are difficult to detect on physical examination as often the peritoneum is not irritated.

## Radiographic examination

Diagnosis of abdominal injuries can be facilitated by a wide variety of investigations, including diagnostic peritoneal lavage (DPL), radiological investigations such as plain radiographs with and without contrast, ultrasonography, radionuclide scanning, angiography, computed tomography, and magnetic resonance imaging.

The specific imaging technique chosen depends on the availability of the modality in the institution as well as the clinical condition of the patient.

# THE TECHNIQUES AVAILABLE

## Conventional radiography

### Initial radiographs

All blunt-trauma patients should have radiographs of the cervical spine, chest, and pelvis performed because these are the investigations most likely to reveal abnormalities requiring an early change in management. Ideally this is done in the resuscitation area with fixed radiographic equipment, but the use of portable radiographic equipment is acceptable. Emergency personnel likely to be exposed to the radiation should be appropriately shielded. The transfer of multiply injured patients to the radiology department for these initial radiographs should be discouraged, as the time wasted and the lack of emergency personnel to accompany the patient may result in an unfavourable outcome. The subsequent radiographic approach for these patients is dictated by their clinical condition.

A supine anteroposterior pelvic radiograph should be obtained if possible, as the clinical diagnosis of pelvic fracture by manual testing is not reliable. The identification of pelvic bony injuries should indicate the potential for severe haemorrhage. Other definitive radiographs can be performed as indicated by the mechanism of injury and results of the secondary survey.

Supine radiographs of the abdomen are not done routinely as part of the initial radiograph series. In penetrating injuries caused by bullets or other projectiles, plain radiographs in two dimensions may be used to locate any foreign bodies. The entrance and exit wounds can be marked with small, radiopaque skin clips to determine the trajectory of the projectile. Radiographs may also be helpful if the projectile has embolized elsewhere.

All unnecessary opaque devices should be removed so as not to interfere with the interpretation, as small pieces of metal may simulate foreign bodies and the creases of any unnecessary clothing or sheets may mimic intrathoracic or intra-abdominal free air. Plain abdominal radiography has a low sensitivity and lacks specificity for identification of abdominal injury. It cannot detect small to moderate quantities of peritoneal fluid or small amounts of free peritoneal air.

Often, the clinical condition of the patient does not allow an erect examination, and if pneumoperitoneum is suspected, the additional view of a right-side-up decubitus examination may provide the required information. The patient can remain on the stretcher in the resuscitation area and the studies performed with portable X-ray equipment. Free air in the peritoneal cavity accumulates along the right lobe of the liver, and again the patient should remain in this position for a few minutes before the examination. The absence of demonstrable pneumoperitoneum on the radiograph does not exclude rupture of a hollow viscus. Small perforations may be self-sealing or be covered by omentum or mesentery, or the amount of free air may be so small as to be undetectable radiographically.

## Radiographic signs in trauma

### Pneumoperitoneum

Pneumoperitoneum is commonly seen in penetrating abdominal or pelvic trauma. In blunt trauma, it occurs when there is a tear in a hollow viscus resulting from a shearing force from sudden deceleration or rupture from a sudden increase in intraluminal pressure. Gross pneumoperitoneum appears radiographically as lucent collections of gas conforming to the inferior surfaces of the diaphragm. However, the radiographic signs of pneumoperitoneum on the supine abdominal film may be subtle. The falciform ligament is outlined when free air is present on both sides of the ligament and appears as a curvilinear density adjacent to the right paravertebral region underlying the liver shadow. The full thickness of the bowel wall is demonstrated when there is free intraperitoneal air outlining the serosal surface of loops that contain intraluminal gas. Free air tends to rise and accumulate in the central abdomen in a supine patient and this may appear as a lucent oval shadow, mimicking the shape of an American football and hence termed the 'football sign'.

A dilated stomach, which often occurs in patients sustaining abdominal trauma, or after cardiopulmonary resuscitation, may obscure the air under the left hemidiaphragm. Occasionally, dilated loops of bowel may radiographically mimic free air or obscure genuine collections entirely. Not all cases of pneumoperitoneum are due to ruptured bowel, other causes including pneumomediastinum and prior diagnostic peritoneal lavage.

### Haemoperitoneum

In patients with significant abdominal injury, haemoperitoneum is a common finding. Blood may initially be localized around the injured organ, contained by the true or false capsule of the involved organ, or distributed freely in the peritoneal cavity. Plain radiographs of the abdomen are not useful for the radiological assessment of haemoperitoneum as they are insensitive and the volume of the free blood must be greater than 800 ml before any classic plain radiographic signs can be demonstrated. By gravitation, the fluid will accumulate in the most dependent part of the abdomen. In the supine patient, this is the intraperitoneal portion of the pelvis and the pouch of Douglas. Accumulation of blood here presents as the classic radiographic finding known as 'dog ears', resulting from blood within the lateral recesses beside the bladder. These appear as soft-tissue densities that project superolaterally to the bladder, with an accompanying thin radiolucent line that follows the contour of the dome of the bladder, produced when extraperitoneal fat is interposed between the blood-filled distended pelvic peritoneum and the urinary bladder.

Other radiological appearances on the supine film include opacification locally or diffusely and widening of the space between the lateral wall of the colon and the radiolucent vertical flank stripe, caused by the displacement of the right or left colon medially by blood collections in the paracolic gutters. However, the radiolucent fat of the flank stripe may be obscured by haematoma or inflammation within the lateral abdominal wall. Because of its mesenteric attachments, small bowel floats toward the centre of the abdomen and a further radiographic sign of haemorrhage may be a generalized ground-glass appearance in other areas of the abdomen.

### Retroperitoneal haemorrhage

Retroperitoneal haemorrhage may result in the obliteration of the lateral psoas or renal shadow and can displace the bladder away from the side of haemorrhage. However, the site of the injury cannot be determined and a normal radiograph does not exclude significant retroperitoneal abdominal injuries.

### Penetrating injuries

Metallic retained foreign bodies or missiles are normally easily identified on plain abdominal radiographs, and any associated skeletal damage can be assessed. Injuries caused by high-velocity bullets often produce a high-energy transfer with fragmentation of the missile and therefore many small foreign bodies may be found. In the absence of an exit wound, a careful search is required for any foreign body that may have bounced to a more distant location, for example into the chest.

## Radionuclide scanning

In the days before the ready availability of CT scans, this modality played an important role in the investigation of abdominal injuries.

There are several drawbacks to the use of this modality. Patients must be haemodynamically stable before they can be transferred to the nuclear medicine department. The presence of resuscitation equipment, such as chest tubes and backboards, may interfere with image acquisition. The scanning of the liver and spleen does not provide information regarding other structures in the abdomen and pelvis and cannot detect any intraperitoneal or retroperitoneal haemorrhage.

The applications of radionuclide scanning are now limited to the following:

1. The use of radionuclide angiography to detect small vascular injuries. For a more sensitive test, a $^{99}Tc^m$-labelled RBC study can be used, and bleeding as little as 1 ml/minute can be diagnosed.

2. Injury to the renal cortex and collecting system, and renal function and perfusion can be assessed by the use of renal scintigraphy using [$^{99}Tc^m$]diethylenetriamine pentaacetic acid, [$^{99}Tc^m$]dimercapto-succinic acid, or [$^{131}I$]hippuran. It can also be used in the period after acute trauma to follow the course of renal function compromised by direct trauma or secondary to acute tubular necrosis.

## Ultrasonography

This modality has been used increasingly in the investigation of abdominal trauma, in place of diagnostic peritoneal lavage (DPL), especially in centres where the A&E personnel are trained to perform this mode of investigation. Its main advantage over DPL is that it can be performed quickly and non-invasively and, should the need arise, it may be repeated to assess any bleeding that is not apparent in the initial scan. Other advantages include equipment portability, no radiation, and the ability to record motion such as vascular pulsation.

Ultrasound is particularly useful in detecting intraperitoneal fluid collections in patients with blunt abdominal trauma. It is a useful alternative initial screening modality in haemodynamically unstable patients whose abdominal examination findings are equivocal or unreliable. These patients cannot always be transferred safely to the CT suite, but bedside ultrasonography can be performed rapidly.

Another application of ultrasound examination is in following the resolution or progression of lesions in patients with established diagnoses.

In the hands of well-trained personnel, the ultrasound diagnosis of haemoperitoneum is as sensitive as DPL. This diagnosis is made by the detection of free fluid in the dependent parts of the abdomen or pelvis. Residual peritoneal lavage fluid cannot be distinguished from haemoperitoneum and it is better to perform the ultrasound examination first. Additional information may be gained from a further examination to seek the cause of the haemoperitoneum, for example, laceration of the liver, spleen, or kidney. These injuries are diagnosed by the presence of subcapsular intraparenchymal haematomas, and the ultrasonographic appearance depends on how long the injury has been present.

Six-view examinations are done for the detection of haemoperitoneum and cardiac tamponade in a multiple-trauma patient, and the areas examined are the hepatorenal recess, splenorenal recess, both paracolic gutters, subdiaphragmatic space, and the pouch of Douglas or retrovesical space. The whole process can be completed quickly without moving the patient.

The use of ultrasound may be limited by abdominal wall injuries and gaseous distension of the stomach and intestine.

## Computed tomography

The increasing availability of the CT scan has made this non-invasive modality an alternative investigation in the evaluation of abdominal trauma. CT offers anatomical views of the entire abdomen, including the pelvic structures and retroperitoneum, with excellent resolution. Skeletal structures, soft tissue, and spinal canal are more clearly delineated by CT than by other imaging modalities.

It is able to demonstrate both intra-abdominal and retroperitoneal structures as well as determining the severity of the injuries. It allows stable injuries to be readily diagnosed and treated conservatively with a period of observation, and laparotomy is then performed only if there is worsening of the haemodynamic status. Other incidental and unsuspected injuries may be demonstrated by CT scanning, it is not limited by the presence of intestinal distension, and does not require a change in patient position.

Although no modality is ideal in the evaluation of abdominal trauma, CT is suitable in haemodynamically stabilized patients who have equivocal physical findings or altered conscious level due to influence of drugs or alcohol. When peritoneal lavage is relatively contraindicated (as in patients who have had multiple previous abdominal surgery, massive obesity, or bleeding diathesis), CT is particularly useful in the evaluation of abdominal injuries.

Important points to consider are the availability of resuscitation equipment in the CT suite and allowance for the continuous monitoring of the patient while CT is being performed.

Many studies have compared CT with other modalities and diagnostic peritoneal lavage in the evaluation of abdominal trauma. The outcome of these studies has varied greatly, and this may well be due to differences in patient selection, the characteristics of the CT scanner, and the level of expertise in performance and interpretation of CT scans in different centres. The optimal use of contrast material and elimination of artefacts are considerations in achieving maximum resolution and in assessing the parenchymal structures accurately in abdominal CT. Intravenous contrast material enhances the attenuation difference between parenchymal organ tissue and haematoma within lacerations, and abdominal vascular structures become well delineated. Enteral contrast material opacifies the intestinal lumen, enhancing the visualization of the gastrointestinal tract, including the bowel wall itself.

By reducing the scanning time, the respiratory motion artefact can be reduced and this may be achieved with a helical CT scanner. To diminish other sources of artefact, objects such as cardiac monitoring leads and intravenous lines should be removed from the scanning field.

CT is highly accurate in detecting solid visceral and retroperitoneal injuries. It has poor sensitivity in the detection of hollow visceral and pancreatic injuries.

In some centres, the CT scan is preferred to diagnostic peritoneal lavage as the initial investigation of choice in abdominal trauma. This also allows angiography to be performed after the CT to assess the rate of bleeding in hepatic and splenic injuries that are treated non-operatively. However, there may be interference from the contrast adminstered for the CT scan.

When peritoneal lavage is used as the initial investigation for abdominal trauma, CT may be used to delineate the organs injured in a stable patient with a positive or equivocal lavage. The problem with this practice is that there may be a false impression of haemoperitoneum when the peritoneal lavage fluid is incompletely removed, as is normally the case.

It is important to scan the entire peritoneal cavity, from the highest hemidiaphragm to below the pubic symphysis, as failure to do so may result in the overlooking of a small collection of free blood in the subphrenic space or pelvis. The slice thickness should be at 10 mm, and sometimes 5 mm slices may be needed to provide better visualization of doubtful areas in the pancreas, duodenum, and adrenal glands. Scanning should be performed with both soft-tissue and bone windows, and lung windows for all upper scans that include the chest and lungs.

## Magnetic resonance imaging

At present, magnetic resonance imaging is not suitable for the initial evaluation of abdominal injuries. It is restricted to stable patients who do not need continuous life-support and monitoring devices, and who are able to co-operate with the examination and remain immobile. MRI plays a part in investigating trauma patients after stabilization. The ability to provide multiplanar imaging is definitely advantageous when specific anatomical detail is needed. For soft-tissue imaging, it provides better visualization than the CT scan.

## Angiography

Angiography has no role as a screening modality in the evaluation of abdominal trauma as it is expensive, time consuming, and invasive.

More importantly, it may be hazardous for unstable patients to be transferred to the angiography suite for radiological examination. One exception would be the embolization of bleeding pelvic vessels in unstable patients with pelvic fracture, where interventional radiology can play a part in therapy.

The reliability of using angiography in the detection of intra-abdominal injuries is not known. The principal application of angiography in abdominal trauma is in the demonstration of ongoing haemorrhage from injured organs and its role in potential simultaneous therapy. It is known that diagnosis of intrarenal and extraperitoneal vascular injuries by physical examination and laboratory studies is difficult, and these injuries commonly result in haemodynamic instability for which evaluation by early angiography may be necessary. In haemodynamically stable patients with confirmed visceral injuries, follow-up angiography is useful to confirm active haemorrhage that may require embolization, suggested by both clinical parameters and falling haematocrit. Angiography may be used to identify major vascular injuries, and selective catheterization and therapeutic embolization of actively bleeding vessels can be done at the same time.

## Contrast studies

Contrast studies have a minor role in the evaluation of abdominal trauma. Oral or enteral contrast may be administered when CT scanning is performed to delineate injuries to a hollow viscus, and water-soluble gastrograffin is helpful in patients with suspected gastric, duodenal, or rectal perforations. All contrast studies may obscure angiography and should be avoided if interventional radiology is likely to be required in the early stages of management.

# IMAGING OF SPECIFIC INJURIES

## Spleen

The spleen is commonly injured in both blunt and penetrating trauma and can follow major or even apparently minor trauma. The possibility of splenic injury should be considered following trauma in which the mechanism of injury involves impact to the left lower thorax or left upper abdomen. The closeness of the spleen to the left lower ribs also makes it vulnerable to injuries when these ribs are fractured. There may be signs of haemorrhagic shock together with generalized peritoneal signs when there is free intraperitoneal blood. Physical findings that may also suggest splenic injury include external signs of left upper quadrant trauma, left lower rib fractures, and left upper quadrant tenderness or rebound. It must be remembered that the absence of these signs does not rule out even severe trauma to the spleen.

Assessment of the use of the various imaging modalities in the initial evaluation of splenic injuries must take into consideration their sensitivity.

## Conventional radiography

The findings on abdominal radiographs are non-specific for splenic injuries and therefore are of limited usefulness. Significant splenic injury may occur without any abnormalities being detected on plain radiographs. Radiographic signs of haemoperitoneum are seen when there is a significant quantity of intraperitoneal blood from splenic disruption. There may be enlargement of the splenic mass due to haematoma, which causes displacement of the gastric air shadow medially and the colon inferiorly at the splenic flexure. The left hemidiaphragm may be elevated.

Signs such as left lower rib fractures and left haemothorax present on the chest radiograph may suggest splenic injuries.

## Radionuclide scanning

The main role of radionuclide scanning in abdominal trauma has been in the detection of liver and splenic injuries. Its limitation, however, is its inability to evaluate injuries to other organs and to identify and quantify free intraperitoneal blood. Splenic defects identified as decreased uptake may represent either normal variants of anatomy, such as clefts, or other non-traumatic splenic defects such as cysts.

## Ultrasonography

In the detection of splenic injuries, ultrasonography is a relatively sensitive modality and is useful as an initial screening tool (Fig. 13.1). The presence of injury is demonstrated by the following features:

(1) haematoma within or adjacent to the spleen;

(2) distortion of the spleen;

(3) perisplenic fluid collection;

(4) displacement of upper abdominal organs by adjacent haematoma.

The echogenicity of a haematoma changes with its age. As the haematoma liquefies, its echogenicity is increased and therefore it

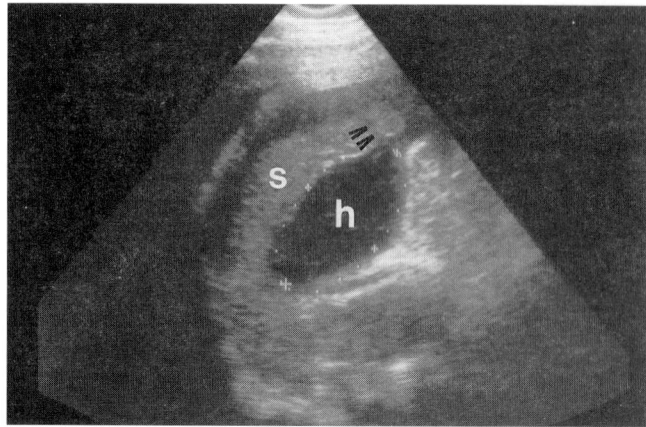

**Fig. 13.1** Ultrasound examination of the spleen. Splenic laceration with surrounding haematoma: >, laceration of s (spleen); h, haematoma.

becomes more easily distinguisable from the normal splenic echo texture. Information regarding the condition of the other organs can be obtained simultaneously.

### Angiography

Angiography is an invasive procedure which is expensive and time consuming and requires a specially trained radiologist. For these reasons, it is not suitable for the initial screening of splenic injuries but rather to clarify situations in which the source of continuous intraperitoneal bleeding cannot be identified by other modalities. The evaluation of other injuries, such as bleeding pelvic vessels from pelvic fractures or renal pedicle disruption, by renal arteriography allows the spleen to be evaluated at the same time.

Embolization of actively bleeding splenic vessels remains an area of controversy, with evidence still being gathered.

### Computed tomography

For the detection of splenic injuries, CT with contrast is a highly sensitive modality, with reported rates of between 96 and 98 per cent (Fig. 13.2). It is able to demonstrate the anatomical detail of the splenic injury as well as detecting injuries to other abdominal organs. CT has also been used to predict the clinical course of patients with splenic injuries and thus the feasibility of treating splenic injuries non-operatively. However, the results vary greatly in different series of patients. When treated non-surgically, follow-up includes a CT examination with contrast, usually repeated 3–5 days later and again at 4–6 weeks after initial assessment in clinically asymptomatic patients.

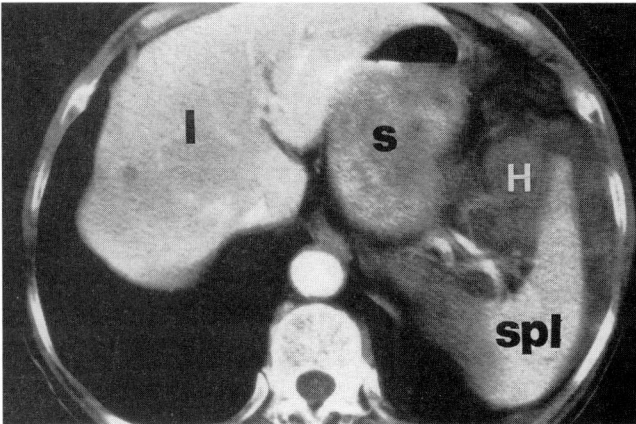

**Fig. 13.2** CT abdomen (contrast), splenic laceration with surrounding haematoma: H, haematoma surrounding the spleen; l, liver; s, stomach; spl, spleen.

Detection of postsplenectomy complications such as haemorrhage, and documentation of resolution of intraperitoneal haemorrhage are some of the other applications of CT.

On a non-enhanced CT, haematoma around or within the spleen is isodense or of higher density in comparison to the intact splenic parenchyma. The detection of splenic injury is optimized by the adminstration of intravenous contrast material which will enhance the splenic parenchyma, making its appearance denser than the adjacent haematoma, splenic contusion, or laceration. Any patchy appearance of splenic-tissue density suggests splenic haematoma coexisting with undamaged parenchyma.

The splenic parenchyma may be indented by subcapsular haematoma, which can have a layered appearance, due to alternating layers of clotted and non-clotted blood within the haematoma. Lacerations are often detected as subtle irregularities or shallow defects in the surface contour of the spleen. When air is seen within the splenic parenchyma, it may be due to subcapsular haematoma complicated by infection, or it may have been introduced by a penetrating injury. The differences in appearance between the injured and normal splenic tissue can be enhanced by varying the CT 'windows'.

## Liver

Injuries to the liver account for a large share of the morbidity and mortality associated with abdominal trauma. The mortality from hepatic injury tends to increase with the number of associated injuries. The location of the liver predisposes it to laceration by overlying fractured rib fragments. The right lobe, constituting 80 per cent of the liver volume, is the most frequent site of injury from both blunt and penetrating forces. Its ligamentous attachments also pre-dispose it to tethering injuries at these fixed points during accelera-tion–deceleration mechanisms.

The evaluation of hepatic injuries must be made in the context of the clinical situation. Patients with uncontrolled haemorrhagic shock must be resuscitated and the injuries treated surgically as soon as pos-sible. In these cases, no imaging is done. In haemodynamically stable patients, more thorough diagnostic assessment could be performed for a more precise definition of the injuries.

Clinical findings in the diagnosis of liver injury are non-specific and usually include signs of haemorrhagic shock due to blood loss and peritoneal irritation. Injuries to the liver should be suspected in the presence of a history or signs of impact over the right lower thorax or right upper abdomen, especially if there is tenderness, guarding, or rebound in the right upper quadrant. Sometimes radiation of pain to the right shoulder or periscapular region may be present.

## Conventional radiography

This is highly unreliable, but some signs when present are suggestive of hepatic injuries. Perihepatic haematoma may manifest radiogra-phically as increased opacification of the right upper quadrant and a shift of bowel shadow away from that region. Fractures of the right lower ribs on the chest or abdominal film may heighten suspicion of the possibility of liver injuries. More sensitive techniques are recom-mended for confirmation of liver injury when this is suspected.

## Ultrasonography

The ultrasonographic evaluation of the liver shares the same advan-tages, limitations, and accuracy as that of ultrasonography of splenic injury. It can demonstrate the presence of minimal amounts of free intraperitoneal fluid, can be performed in the resuscitation area without moving the patient, and can demonstrate solid-organ injuries with high resolution. Again, there are factors limiting its use, includ-ing bowel gas obscuring the underlying anatomy and dependence on the skill of the operator. With increasing availability of the ultrasound machine, this modality is proving to be an excellent screening device in the detection of solid organ-injuries. The features of hepatic injuries are similar to those of other solid-organ injuries and appear as follows:

1.  Lacerations appear as anechoic defects. As the blood clots, the laceration may appear echogenic.

2.  Haematomas are seen as anechoic collections with a slight distal acoustic enhancement initially, and become echogenic as blood

begins to clot. In the later stages, liquefaction of the clot occurs and the appearance is complex or cystic.

3. Subcapsular haematomas appear anechoic and become more complex later depending on the stage of clotting and resorption. Occasionally, fluid–debris and fluid–fluid levels may be seen within the resolving haematomas.

## Radionuclide scanning

The use of radionuclide scanning using technetium has largely been replaced by other modalities which are more accurate, faster, and accessible. It provides poor anatomical detail and does not demonstrate the cause of any defects that are detected. Positive findings are similar to those discussed under injuries to the spleen.

## Angiography

Angiography detects the presence of liver injury accurately and, when indicated, has the added advantage of allowing therapeutic embolization of any vessels involved in haemorrhage.

## Computed tomography

CT has been used increasingly in the diagnosis of solid-organ injuries, especially in diagnosing and guiding the management of blunt trauma to the liver. Its sensitivity and specificity is comparable to that of peritoneal lavage, but it is also able to provide anatomical delineation of the injuries. It demonstrates all types of injuries, including contusions, subcapsular and intraparenchymal haematomas, lacerations, fractures, and major crush and parenchymal avulsion injuries, as well as devascularization and haemorrhage within or around the gallbladder.

CT can serve as a guide for the planning of surgical approaches in both blunt and penetrating injury. Again, as with splenic injuries, serial CT studies after initial injury can provide follow-up for assessment of healing or for the detection of complications such as biloma, delayed bleeding, or abscess formation.

Four basic types of injuries are recognized by CT: lacerations, haematomas, fragmentation, and periportal blood tracking.

Lacerations may be superficial or deep. Superficial lacerations are arbitrarily defined as those extending less than 3 cm from the surface. Lacerations may be isolated or may merge into areas of contusion or haematoma. Compressive forces from blunt trauma may result in a typical pattern of parallel linear lacerations radiating out from the hilar region, a pattern with radiating , parallel, and jagged borders known as the 'bear claw'.

Parenchymal haematoma generally appears on CT as a central high-density area of clotted blood surrounded by lower-density, non-clotted blood or an area of contusion. With time, haematomas show a gradual decrease in attenuation to the extent of their mimicking the appearance of water.

Fragments of the liver may be completely avulsed, or the vascular supply to some segments may be cut off by proximal injuries to the perihilar area. During contrast CT, these segments will fail to enhance with the rest of the liver and appear as wedge-shaped unenhanced areas that extend to the periphery.

Periportal blood tracking is sometimes seen in blunt liver injuries and consists of areas of low-attenuation density paralleling the portal venous tracts. This is attributed to haemorrhage tracking along the periportal connective tissue.

Penetrating injuries to the hepatobiliary system are generally explored surgically, and in haemodynamically stable patients the role of CT would be to guide this process by defining the extent of the injuries and their proximity to the hilum and other adjacent structures.

Some surgical series have demonstrated that 50–70 per cent of hepatic injuries are not bleeding at the time of laparotomy. Increasing numbers of blunt liver injuries are being treated non-surgically in haemodynamically stable patients, and CT has a role to play in this group of patients. This trend of using CT to guide non-operative treatment was first used in children and is less well established in adults. The prerequisites for such management are the easy access and availability of CT scans, and personnel with experience in the interpretation of trauma CT should be readily available for consultation. Ward facilities, including experienced staff for close monitoring, should also be available and if deterioration occurs, follow-up CT scanning, operating facilities, and experienced surgical and anaesthesia staff should be readily available.

## Pancreas

The pancreas is one of the least commonly injured solid viscera, and it is uncommon for patients to sustain isolated injuries to the pancreas, due to the relatively well-protected site. Diagnosis of pancreatic injury is usually made at laparotomy performed for management of other associated abdominal injuries.

In blunt trauma, injuries to the neck region of the pancreas are more common, as this is likely to be compressed directly between the vertebral column and the force applied externally. In adults, this is usually a steering wheel in motor vehicle accidents and in children, direct compression by the handlebars of a bicycle, or by being run over by a motor vehicle. The mortality rate in pancreatic trauma increases with the number of other associated injuries and is greatly increased when there is coexistent rupture of either the duodenum or colon. Complications of pancreatic injuries include pancreatic fistula, intra-abdominal abscess, and pseudocyst formation, and the rate of these increases when the diagnosis is delayed.

Initially, severe pancreatic injury may be clinically silent, evolving only slowly over a period of hours to days, but symptoms are relatively non-specific and may be masked by other associated injuries. There may be moderate to severe constant epigastic pain with radiation to the back, and associated symptoms of nausea, vomiting, and anorexia. The clinical signs range from mild tenderness at the epigastrium to frank generalized peritonitis and shock.

The measurement of serum amylase and diagnostic peritoneal lavage have been used in the detection of pancreatic injuries. A single measurement of serum amylase is not reliable in pancreatic trauma. Persistently increased or rising serum amylase measurements are more specific but are of limited usefulness in the emergency setting.

The radiographic approach to the diagnosis of pancreatic injury is limited.

**Conventional radiography**

The findings on conventional radiographs are non-specific (Table 13.1).

**Ultrasonography**

This is useful in the assessment of the acutely traumatized pancreas but the limitations are similar to those in the evaluation of other abdominal organs.

Signs of injury include focal oedema or frank pancreatic disruption, haematoma around the pancreas, and retroperitoneal haemorrhage.

**Computed tomography**

There is considerable controversy in the role of CT in pancreatic injuries. Some investigators have shown a high incidence of false-positive results, thereby raising the question of its accuracy.

**Table 13.1** Radiographic features suggestive of pancreatic injury

| Pancreatic causes | Radiographic signs |
| --- | --- |
| Localized ileus overlying epigastric area | Sentinel loops of bowel |
| Pancreatic haematoma | Widening of the sweep of the duodenum and displacement of the stomach and hollow viscera |
| Ascites | Generalized haziness of the abdomen |

Signs of injury depend on the severity of the injuries. Pancreatic fracture may be diagnosed by the separation of the two ends of the gland by fluid in the prerenal space. A contused pancreas may appear to be focally or diffusely enlarged and shows areas of decreased attenuation. However, the signs are often subtle and include peripancreatic fluid collections or haemorrhage.

False-positive results occur as a result of:

(1) technical problems such as motion artefact;

(2) adjacent bowel loops mimicking the appearance of peripancreatic haematoma;

(3) fluid or blood in the lesser sac;

(4) injuries of other abdominal organs giving rise to haematoma around the pancreas.

Follow up CT is also useful in detecting complications of pancreatic injury, which include fistulae, abscesses, pseudocysts, and pancreatitis.

### Endoscopic retrograde cholangiopancreatography (ERCP)

ERCP is an imaging modality which can evaluate the integrity of the ductal system. The presence of post-traumatic stricture is the main cause of recurrent pancreatitis. This investigation is suitable for stable patients with incompletely determined signs of pancreatic injury, rather than as a primary diagnostic tool.

## Hollow viscera

Injuries to the hollow viscera are more common after penetrating trauma and are often multiple. In blunt trauma, a major contributing mechanism is the incorrect wearing of seat belts in victims of motor vehicular accidents, and the most frequently injured portion of the small bowel is the duodenum.

Clinical diagnosis is often difficult, especially in blunt trauma. Signs of abdominal tenderness, rigidity, and absent bowel sounds are often not found. In small bowel injury, bleeding is often not severe and the light bacterial load results in spillage that is less irritating, and signs of peritonitis may appear late. In stomach perforation with an acid fluid pH, and the large intestinal perforation with a heavy bacterial load, earlier symptoms may result. Delay in diagnosis and treatment increase the morbidity and mortality and this is especially dramatic if repair is delayed beyond 24 hours.

Mesenteric vessel injuries are often rapidly fatal and patients who survive to reach the emergency department are often critically unstable. The majority of these patients are taken directly to surgery without further diagnostic procedures, and indications for angiography are, in any case, difficult to identify preoperatively.

## Conventional radiography

This modality is relatively insensitive in detecting hollow visceral injuries and findings are non-specific. Perforation or rupture may not always produce intraperitoneal or retroperitoneal free air in the early stages. The small intestine contains little gas and detection of pneumoperitoneum is difficult on plain radiographs (Fig. 13.3). In order to detect small amounts of free air, optimal positioning, such as in the erect or lateral decubitus position, is required and this is often not possible in a multiply injured patient. Additional associated signs on abdominal radiographs include the 'double wall' sign, in which the free intraperitoneal and intraluminal gas outline both sides of the bowel wall, making it clearly visible on the plain films .

Obliteration of the psoas muscles and the presence of stippled air bubbles outlining the psoas muscles, kidneys, or pancreas suggest rupture of retroperitoneal hollow viscera. Retroperitoneal free air is particularly difficult to detect.

## Contrast studies

In stable patients, studies using water-soluble contrast material such as gastrograffin are useful in the diagnosis of perforation. Besides extravasation of contrast, other signs include obstruction due to the presence of an intramural haematoma.

Water-soluble contrast enema with fluoroscopy remains the optimal test to evaluate colon perforation.

## Computed tomography

CT is not sensitive in detecting isolated bowel injuries and is of limited value. In penetrating injuries where there is a high incidence of associated bowel injury, CT should not be used as the only diagnostic modality.

Radiological signs include free peritoneal fluid and air, mesenteric infiltration, thickened bowel wall, and the presence of sentinel clot (focal accumulation of clotted blood adjacent to the injured bowel). In many patients who have sustained significant abdominal injuries, administration of oral or rectal water-soluble contrast to opacify the bowel is not possible.

# Genitourinary system

In general, the management of life-threatening injuries takes precedence over that of urological injuries. Unfortunately the diagnostic

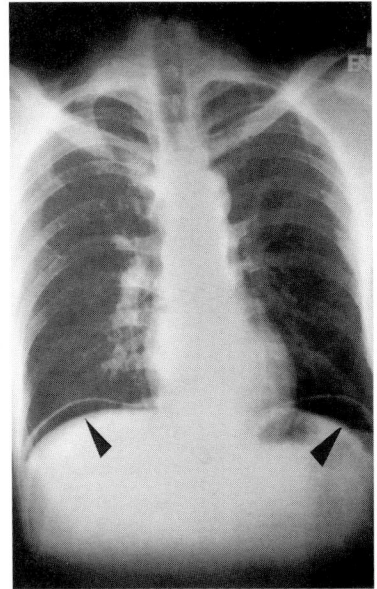

**Fig. 13.3** Chest, erect frontal view: ◄, pneumoperitoneum—free gas under the diaphragm.

evaluation of genitourinary trauma may be delayed in such cases, increasing the risk of complications.

The presence of congenital abnormalities such as horseshoe and polycystic kidneys is associated with a higher risk of injuries following trauma. Renal injuries are more common in children and may be due to the relatively scanty perinephric fat and overlying musculature.

In the management of genitourinary injuries, although the history of the mechanism and physical assessment are important, radiological examination is often needed to arrive at a definitive diagnosis, as signs of urinary-tract injury can be subtle. Haematuria by itself has a poor correlation with the injury severity. However, the presence of contusions or abrasions over the flanks or lower abdomen, lower rib fractures, pelvic fracture, perineal swelling or scrotal haematoma, and abdominal tenderness should raise the suspicion of renal or urinary-tract injuries.

## Kidney injuries

The kidneys are commonly injured in both penetrating and blunt abdominal trauma. Penetrating injuries of the flank are explored operatively because of the high incidence of associated injuries to the adjacent bowel, liver, or spleen.

### The classification of renal injury

There is no universally accepted classification system for renal trauma, but a functional classification has been devised that applies to both blunt and penetrating trauma. Penetrating injuries are more often associated with the major and catastrophic categories.

Minor (majority of cases):

- minor laceration

- renal contusion

- intrarenal haematoma

- segmental infarction

- small subcapsular haematoma.

Major:

- parenchymal laceration extending to and communicating with the collecting system

- large subcapsular haematoma

- complete laceration

- renal vein injury.

Catastrophic:

- shattered kidney—fragmentation (which accounts for 1 per cent of renal injuries)

- renal artery avulsion or occlusion (often associated with blunt trauma).

### Diagnostic imaging

*Intravenous pyelogram (IVP)*   The indications for IVP are controversial. Computed tomography (CT) has largely replaced its use in patients with potential renal trauma since CT allows all organs in the upper abdomen and retroperitoneal structures to be evaluated at the same time. IVP is used in centres where CT is not readily available, or when the injured patient is too unstable to be moved, in which case a bedside 7-minute IVP can be performed.

*Computed tomography (CT)*   CT allows the accurate assessment of the presence and extent of renal injury and any associated adjacent organ injuries. The use of helical (spiral) CT reduces the investigation time needed and imaging of the abdomen currently needs as little as 20–30 seconds. It also enables follow-up assessment to be performed easily. The advent of CT has allowed more conservative modes of treatment and reduced the incidence of surgical intervention.

*Ultrasonography*   Although renal ultrasonography can be performed at the bedside, it is not always useful in the emergency setting. The kidneys, being retroperitoneal structures, are difficult to evaluate in the supine patient as their views are commonly obscured by dilated bowel caused by ileus. It is, however, useful as a follow-up study in the detection of urinoma and haematoma of the kidney.

*Renal angiography*   Selective renal angiography is useful in patients sustaining blunt renal injury with expanding large perirenal or retroperitoneal haematoma. In such cases, the bleeding vessel can be identified and embolized, sometimes sparing the patient the need for surgery and general anaesthesia.

Injuries to the renal vascular pedicle usually occur in severe trauma and often the patient arrives at the Accident and Emergency department exsanguinated and requires immediate surgery. Angiography is therefore not commonly performed.

### Ureter and bladder

The ureters are well protected in the retroperitoneal space and therefore they are rarely injured. Injuries that do occur are often associated with penetrating stab or projectile trauma. In children hyperextension injuries to the lumbar spine may lead to disruption at the pelvic–ureteric junction. Although rare, missed ureteric injuries can result in renal failure when fibrosis and stricture occur.

Bladder injuries often occur in association with pelvic fractures, due to their close anatomical relationship. Injuries occur more often when the bladder is full and range from simple contusion to frank rupture. In a conscious patient with bladder injuries, there is lower abdominal pain, haematuria or inability to void, and abdominal distension.

Rupture of the bladder can be either intraperitoneal or extraperitoneal. Intraperitoneal rupture often occurs as a result of a deceleration injury to the lower abdomen or pelvis when the bladder is full. Extraperitoneal rupture may occur with laceration from a bony fragment as a result of pelvic fracture.

**Diagnostic imaging**

### KUB (kidney, ureter, bladder) plain radiograph

KUB is often used in the initial evaluation of abdominal trauma. About 15 per cent of patients with pelvic fractures have bladder trauma, and 70 per cent of those with bladder rupture have a pelvic fracture.

### Intravenous urogram (IVU)

This investigation often obviates the need for other imaging modalities in the evaluation of ureteric injuries. A negative IVU does not rule out the presence of bladder rupture, and if there is a strong clinical suspicion, retrograde cystography is indicated.

### Computed tomography

CT of the pelvis may be performed for direct indications or as part of the evaluation of abdominal trauma. An advantage of CT is that the patient need not be turned during the study.

**Urethra**

Injuries are seldom life threatening and are found more commonly in males. Typical signs include blood at the urethral meatus (80–90 per cent), scrotal haematoma, perineal swelling, or a high-riding (mobile) prostate on rectal examination. Urethral catherization should not be attempted routinely by inexperienced staff if any of these signs are present.

In the male, posterior urethral injury is often associated with pelvic fracture, whereas injuries to the anterior urethra commonly result from direct trauma crushing the urethra. In the female, urethral injuries most often result from a direct blow to the perineum.

The urethra may be contused or ruptured, and in either case there is frequently blood visible at the external urinary meatus. A retrograde urethrogram is needed to reveal the presence of partial or complete urethral rupture. In urethral injuries, the urinary system should be decompressed before repair is performed, if necessary with suprapubic catheterization.

## Testicular injuries

Traumatic injury to the testes frequently occur from assault, contact sports, and cycling injuries. The mechanism is often a direct blow with compression of the testis against the symphysis pubis. The injury presents as either contusion or rupture. The imaging modality of choice is ultrasonography as it is convenient, comfortable, involves no ionizing radiation, and provides a fairly accurate diagnosis. Colour-flow Doppler ultrasound provides added information regarding alterations in the blood flow of the testes and spermatic cords.

# BIBLIOGRAPHY

Ballinger PW. Merrill's Atlas of Radiographic Positions and Radiologic Procedures, 8th edn. Missouri: Mosby, 1995; 2:31–214.

Basmajian JV. Grant's Method of Anatomy, 11th edn. Baltimore: Williams & Wilkins, 1989.

Cerise EJ, Scully JH Jr. Blunt trauma to the small intestine. J Trauma 1970; 10(1):46–50.

Chandhoke PS, McAninch JW. Detection and significance of microscopic haematuria in patients with blunt renal trauma. J Urol 1988; 140:16.

Cox EF. Blunt abdominal trauma. Ann Surg 1984; 199:467–74.

Dunnick NR, McCallum RW, Sandler CM. Textbook of Uroradiology. Baltimore: Williams & Wilkins, 1991.

Esposito TJ, Gens DR, Smith LG, Scorpio R. Evaluation of blunt abdominal trauma occurring during pregnancy. J Trauma 1989; 29:1628–32.

Fanney DR, Castillas J, Murphy BJ. CT in the diagnosis of renal trauma. Radiographics 1990; 10:29–40.

Federle MP. Computed tomography in blunt abdominal trauma. Radiol Clin North Am 1983; 21(3):461–75.

Federle MP, Kaiser JA, McAninch JW, *et al*. The role of computed tomography in renal trauma. Radiology 1981; 141:455–60.

Guerriero WG. Genitourinary trauma. In: Guerriero WG, ed. Problems in Urology. Philadelphia: JB Lippincott, 1988; 2:186–7.

Jeffrey RB, Federle MP, Crass RA. Computed tomography of pancreatic trauma. Radiology 1983; 147:491–4.

Jeffrey RB, Laing FC, Hriack H, *et al*. Sonography of testicular trauma. AJR 1983; 141:993–5.

Jeffrey RB, Laing FC, Wing VW. Ultrasound in acute pancreatic trauma. Gastrointest Radiol 1986; 11:44–6.

Jones TK, Walsh JW, Maull KL. Diagnostic imaging in blunt trauma of the abdomen. Surg Gynecol Obstet 1983; 157:389–98.

Kisa E, Schenk WG. Indications for emergency intravenous pyelography (IVP) in blunt abdominal trauma: a re-appraisal. J Trauma 1986; 26:1086–9.

Kriegshauser JS, Carrol BA. The urinary tract. In: Rumack CM, Wilson SR, Charboneau JW, eds. Diagnostic Ultrasound. St Louis: Mosby Year Book, 1991.

Levine MS, Scheiner JD, Rubesin SE, et al. Diagnosis of pneumoperitoneum on supine abdominal radiographs. AJR 1991; 156:731–5.

McCort JJ. Splenic trauma. In: McCort JJ, ed. Trauma Radiology. New York: Churchill Livingstone, 1990.

Meschan IA. An Atlas of Anatomy Basic to Radiology. Philadelphia: WB Saunders, 1975.

Mindelzun RE. Liver trauma. In: McCort JJ, ed. Trauma Radiology. New York: Churchill Livingstone, 1990.

Mirrvis SE, Whitley NO, Vainwright JR, Gens DR. Blunt hepatic trauma in adults: CT based classification and correlation with prognosis and treatment. Radiology 1989; 171:27–32.

Mitchell JP. Trauma to the urinary tract. N Engl J Med 1973; 228:90.

Moon Kl, Federle MD. Computed tomography in hepatic trauma. AJR 1983; 141:309–14.

Paul L, Juhl JHF. The Essentials of Roentgen Interpretation, 3rd edn. New York: Harper and Row, 1972.

Pollack HM, Wein AJ. Imaging on renal trauma. Radiology 1989; 172:297–308.

Sandler CM, Philips JM, Harris JD, Toombs BD. Radiology of the bladder and urethra in blunt pelvic trauma. Radiol Clin North Am 1981; 19(1):195–211.

Sciafani SJA, Becker JA. Radiological diagnosis of renal trauma. Urol Radiol 1985; 7:192–200.

Spirnak JP. Pelvic fracture and injury of the lower urinary tract. Surg Clin North Am 1988; 68(5):1057–69.

Stalker HP, Kaufman RA, Towbin R. Patterns of liver injury in childhood: CT analysis. AJR 1986; 147:1199–205.

Tovee EV. Blunt abdominal trauma. J Trauma 1970; 10:72.

Wessells H, McAninch JW. Update on upper urinary tract trauma. AUA update series 1996; 15:110.

# CHAPTER 14

# *The pelvis*

.....................................................................................................................................................................

- Key points: pelvis
- Clinical anatomy
- The techniques available
- Imaging of specific conditions
- Bibliography

---

### Key points: pelvis

1. All major blunt-trauma patients should be suspected of potentially having sustained pelvic fractures.

2. Pelvic fractures are a common cause of occult blood loss and there is a high mortality in those patients with hypovolaemic shock.

3. Plain radiographs play a key role in the initial assessment of pelvic fractures, and primary classification relies on this modality.

4. Pelvic fractures may also involve injuries to nerves, bowel, ureters, bladder, urethra, and uterus. Early identification of injuries to these structures often helps to prevent subsequent complications.

5. The number and seriousness of the associated injuries is directly proportional to the severity of the pelvic fracture.

6. CT is useful in assessing pelvic injuries, and the abdomen may be assessed during the same examination.

---

## CLINICAL ANATOMY

The sacrum and the two innominate bones form the pelvis, which is arranged as a ring-like structure together with the strong ligaments which maintain pelvic stability. The bony pelvis protects the pelvic viscera, transmits the upper body weight to the lower extremities, and provides sites of attachment for the muscles of the trunk and lower extremities.

The innominate bone consists of three parts, namely the ilium, pubis, and ischium. Together these three parts converge to form the acetabulum, a socket that articulates with the head of femur.

The ilia articulate with the sacrum posteriorly at the sacroiliac joints and are held together by strong ligaments. Normally the sacroiliac joints are approximately 2–4 mm in width.

The branches of the internal iliac vessels and lumbosacral nerve plexus are very close to the bony structures and are prone to injury should the adjacent bones be fractured.

Anteriorly, the pubic bones unite at the pubic symphysis but this articulation adds relatively little to the overall stability of the pelvis. The symphysis pubis is normally no more than 5 mm in width. The bladder and the urethra lie just posterior to the pubic symphysis and are vulnerable to injury in fractures involving this region.

The sacrum is a triangular bone which forms the posterior part of the pelvis, consisting of a body and the lateral masses. The coccyx is made up of rudimentary vertebrae and articulates with the inferior part of the sacrum. Coccygeal angulation may be as great as 90° and this can still be within normal limits.

The female pelvis is broader, shallower, and lighter than the male pelvis. In addition, the female pelvic inlet is larger and has a more rounded configuration. The sacrum is wider and curves more sharply posteriorly.

Pelvic fractures constitute about 3 per cent of all skeletal fractures presenting to Accident and Emergency departments. The importance of pelvic fractures lies mainly in the fact that they are associated with high rates of complications and mortality. Mortality from pelvic fractures ranges from 6 to 50 per cent, depending on severity, being especially high in those with hypotension. It is wise to assume that all trauma patient who are victims of blunt multiple trauma or who are unconscious have sustained pelvic fractures.

# THE TECHNIQUES AVAILABLE

## Conventional radiography

### Views to order

Radiography plays an important role in the assessment of pelvic trauma. The physical signs of pelvic injury may not always be obvious or reliable and thus a radiographic examination is often required to establish the diagnosis. However, stabilization of the patient takes priority over obtaining a complete set of radiographic images of the pelvis. Often, an initial simple A-P view is of most use in making management decisions.

In a patient with a pelvic fracture, stabilization of the pelvis is essential as unnecessary movement may aggravate the injury or cause more bleeding. In addition, it is also necessary to prevent secondary intra-abdominal, retroperitoneal, gynaecological, and urological injuries.

The anteroposterior projection of the pelvis should include the entire pelvis along with the proximal femora (Fig. 14.1).

A number of pelvic films taken at the resuscitation room will be often be less than perfect due to the superimposition of faeces, air, and foreign matter, which may obscure bony structures. Therefore, care must be taken when interpreting the radiograph and a high index of suspicion maintained.

Other additional views should be obtained only when the patient is stable. These include lateral, inlet (caudad), and outlet (cephalad) views of the pelvis. A lateral projection should include the lumbosacral junction, sacrum, coccyx, superimposed hip bones, and the upper femur.

The inlet and outlet views are also known as angled views, which can be performed without the need to reposition the patient in the resuscitation room. These views are helpful in delineating the extent of the pelvic fractures and joint disruptions. The inlet view is better in demonstrating the orientation of any pubic ramus fractures and is the single best view to demonstrate the orientation of ilium fractures at the sacroiliac joint. The outlet views are best used to demonstrate

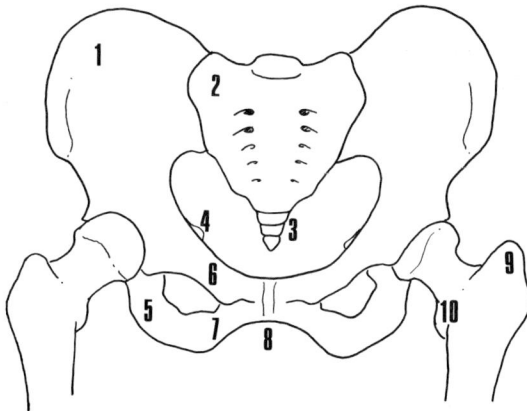

**Fig. 14.1**  Pelvis, anteroposterior view: 1, ilium; 2, sacrum; 3, coccyx; 4, ischial spine; 5, ischium; 6, superior pubic ramus; 7, inferior pubic ramus; 8, pubic symphysis; 9, greater trochanter; 10, lesser trochanter.

the sacrum and sacroiliac joint. In addition they are particularly useful in evaluating the degree of vertical displacement in the fracture fragments or disrupted components of the sacroiliac joint.

Oblique views are often not obtained in the initial period. They can be obtained with the patient in the supine or prone position but the patient may have to be repositioned such that either hip may be elevated. This view provides an excellent assessment of the posterior margin of the acetabulum as well as the relationship between the femoral head and the acetabulum. Oblique views are helpful in the evaluation of acetabular fractures and fracture–dislocation of the hip joint.

## Angiography and interventional radiology

Angiography may be necessary to determine the source of bleeding from pelvic injuries and, possibly, embolization may be used to control bleeding. CT and other special contrast studies, such as micturating cystogram or retrograde urethrogram, may be used in the evaluation of any associated injuries.

# IMAGING OF SPECIFIC CONDITIONS

## Pelvic fractures

### Classification

Fractures of the pelvis are classified by both their stability and the direction of force (mechanism of injury). Stability of the pelvis depends to a great extent on a combination of bones and the integrity of the supporting ligaments, and, in general, the greater the disruption, the greater the degree of instability. Stability of a fracture does not rule out significant soft-tissue injuries, although unstable fractures are more likely to be associated with greater damage. In some cases radiography cannot ascertain whether a fracture is stable and manual manipulation would be needed to elicit motion of the involved hemipelvis. Repeated testing of this nature should be discouraged as movement may worsen the haemorrhage.

Stable fractures include avulsion or chip fractures, single fractures of the pelvic ring, pure acetabular fractures, and straddle fractures of the pubic rami. These account for two-thirds of all pelvic fractures and commonly occur due to low energy transfer motor vehicle accidents, floor-level falls, and recreational or sporting accidents.

Unstable fractures include fractures with two or more breaks in the pelvic ring, such as Malgaigne's fractures (double vertical shearing pelvic injuries), bucket-handle fractures, and open-book fractures (Fig. 14.2). These generally result from accidents involving a greater amount of force, and commonly occur from high-energy motor vehicle accidents, automobile–pedestrian accidents, industrial accidents, and falls from height.

In cases of fractures involving both the superior and inferior rami with a wide degree of displacement, there is increased likelihood of a fracture or disruption posteriorly, and an avulsion fracture of the fifth transverse process is an important clue to the presence of such disruption. Pelvic dislocation is a combination of separation or diastasis of the symphysis pubis and separation of one or both sacroiliac joints.

Open pelvic fractures occur when there is direct communication with the vagina, rectum, or externally through a deep laceration of the skin. When there is air present within the soft tissue around a pelvic fracture on a plain radiograph, the diagnosis may be suspected. Open pelvic fractures are often associated with the subsequent development of retroperitoneal abscess. Mortality in open fractures can be as high as 50 per cent.

Acetabular fractures account for 20 per cent of all pelvic fractures and occur most often from motor vehicle accidents. They are frequently associated with pelvic ring injury. Two-thirds of acetabular fractures are a result of a blow to the greater trochanter or side of the pelvis that forces the acetabulum against the fixed femoral head. The

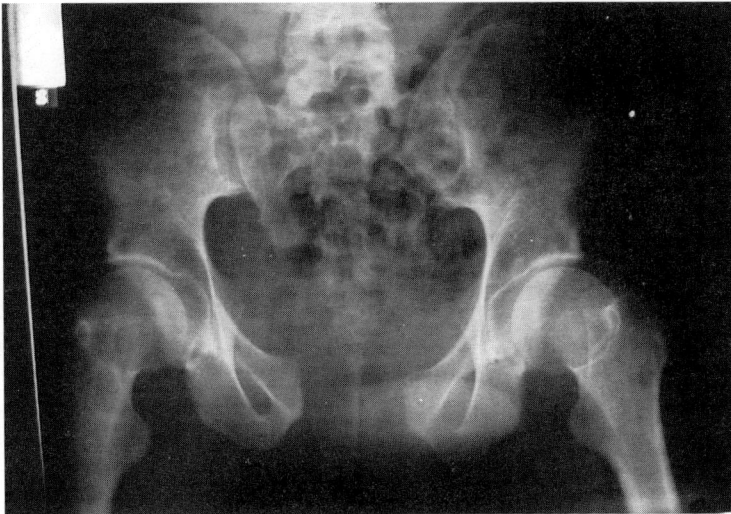

**Fig. 14.2** Pelvis, anteroposterior view. Open-book fracture of the pelvis, an unstable fracture. Note the disrupted symphysis pubis and right sacroiliac joint, and an avulsion fracture of the fifth lumbar transverse process.

**Table 14.1**  Classification of pelvic fractures

| Type | Features |
|------|----------|
| I | Fractures of individual bones without a break in the pelvic ring |
|   | Fractures are usually stable |
|   | Heal well with bed rest |
| II | Single fractures across the pelvic ring |
|   | Fractures are generally stable with little or no displacement |
|   | Are often treated with bed rest |
|   | 25% have associated major soft-tissue and visceral injuries |
| III | Double breaks in the pelvic ring |
|   | Fractures are often unstable |
|   | Frequently associated with soft-tissue and visceral injuries |
| IV | Acetabular fractures |
|   | Often associated with other pelvic injuries |

other third consist of posterior rim fractures that may or may not be associated with posterior dislocation of the hip. Oblique views are often necessary for the evaluation of acetabular fractures, which commonly do not show on the anteroposterior view. Often CT is required to demonstrate the components of the acetabular fracture and location of the femoral head. Other pelvic fractures or fracture–dislocations can also be evaluated accurately using CT and, with multiplanar reconstruction technique, horizontal or transverse fractures of the acetabulum can be demonstrated. This information may be useful in planning subsequent surgical management.

Many classification systems have been proposed for pelvic fractures and many have merits. One example is Kane's adaptation of Key and Conwell's classification, dividing pelvic fractures into four types (Table 14.1).

Pelvic injuries can also be classified by the mechanism of injury and, in particular, the pattern of force. These include anteroposterior compression, lateral compression, vertical shear, and complex (combination) patterns. The most common mechanism of injury is lateral compression.

### Anteroposterior compression fractures

These commonly result from a blow to the front of the pelvis, which gives rise to a range of injuries depending on the amount of force applied. These include vertical fractures of the pubic rami or disruption of the pubic symphysis, open-book fracture or sprung pelvis with external rotation of the iliac wings, and complete separation of the pelvic wings from the sacrum with total disruption of the sacroiliac joint. The mechanism may also include an anteroposterior force which pushes the flexed femur backwards, leading to fracture of the posterior margin of the acetabular rim. Such a mechanism can occur in a motor vehicle accident, particularly affecting unrestrained car drivers and motorcyclists.

Disruption of the sacroiliac joint may not be appreciated on the anteroposterior view of the pelvis, especially when the sacroiliac joint is not widely separated or when the iliac wing is displaced posteriorly. An inlet view of the pelvis would be able to confirm the posterior displacement of the iliac wing.

Associated soft-tissue injuries, including injuries to the bladder and urethra, may occur with fractures of all four rami from a direct anterior compression force.

### *Lateral compression fractures*

The force of injury is from the side and may cause fractures of the pubic rami (100 per cent), sacrum (88 per cent), iliac wing (19 per cent), and quadrilateral plate of the acetabulum with central hip dislocation (19 per cent).

Characteristic features include compression fracture of the ala of the sacrum, a horizontal fracture or buckle fracture of the pubic rami, and fractures of the medial wall of the acetabulum (with or without central hip dislocation). The fracture pattern in reality depends largely on the position along the lateral aspect of the pelvis where the damaging force is applied. The force may be directed anterolaterally or posterolaterally in different circumstances.

Compression fractures of the sacral alae without vertical displacement can be difficult to appreciate on the anteroposterior pelvic radiograph. Careful inspection of the sacral foraminae, including their alignment, can demonstrate the presence of a fracture. Horizontally orientated fractures are easily identified on the anteroposterior view but the presence of coronal fractures can best be demonstrated on the inlet view. Elastic recoil may result in some degree of spontaneous reduction of the displacement, such as in the sacroiliac joints. Fortunately, CT can identify these injuries readily.

These fractures are often associated with paralytic ileus and abdominal guarding, which makes the diagnosis of associated visceral injury difficult clinically.

### *Vertical shear*

This type of injury results in gross pelvic instability. The most common cause is falling or jumping from a height but it may also occur in unrestrained passengers in an automobile accident. The injuring force is usually applied to one or both sides of the pelvis lateral to the midline in an upward direction. The injury includes either fracture of the sacrum or adjacent medial aspect of the iliac wings, or a total tear of all the sacroiliac ligaments on the affected side as well as the disruption of the ligaments of the pubic symphysis. The vertical displacement is usually easily appreciated on the anteroposterior view, but may be reduced in a patient who has had traction applied.

This injury type is associated with calcaneal fractures, compression fractures of the lumbar vertebral bodies, and fractures of the acetabular roof, which are to be expected in view of the mechanism of injury.

### Complex pattern

This pattern occurs when two or more fracture forces are applied, resulting in a combination of injuries and a mixed fracture pattern. This category of injury often involves the acetabulum. CT is usually needed to evaluate the fractures and their associated visceral injuries adequately.

### Computed tomography

Fortunately clinical examination and plain radiographs are sufficient to detect the majority of pelvic-ring disruptions in the acute stage. However, CT is without doubt superior to plain radiographs in obtaining specific detail of sacral fractures, fractures of the acetabular roof, posterior acetabular wall, and quadrilateral plate and sacroiliac joint disruptions. In addition fractures of the hip, loose bodies within the joint, and abnormalities of the soft tissues can also be assessed. Plain radiographs tend to underestimate the extent of injuries, and details of bony injuries may be obscured by the presence of haematoma.

The majority of patients with severe pelvic fractures and major acetabular fractures who are haemodynamically stable will benefit from a CT evaluation of the pelvis.

Multiplanar reconstruction together with three-dimensional reconstruction may be used not only to gain understanding of the fracture anatomy but also to assist in the surgical management of the patient. These reconstructions provide the spatial relationships of the fracture and its fragments. They eliminate superimposed foreign matter, air, and faeces that may otherwise be seen as obscuring artefact. In addition, CT is useful in confirming postoperative reduction.

The necessity to move and reposition the patient to the CT suite means that CT has a limited role in the immediate evaluation of the acutely injured pelvis, except in those centres where a scanner is located within the A&E department with full resuscitation facilities present.

### Pelvic angiography

Injuries to the large pelvic vessels occur in about 2 per cent of all pelvic fractures, and the major cause of death associated with pelvic trauma is haemorrhage. Death rates have been reported to be as high as 60 per cent. In cases when the emergency application of a pelvic external fixator fails to diminish blood loss, pelvic angiography may be valuable in the identification of the bleeding sites that are amenable to percutaneous embolization. In addition, other major abdominal vessels may also be evaluated at the same time. Timely angiography and embolization in cases of traumatic arterial haemorrhage in the pelvis can ultimately help reduce the morbidity and mortality rate, and in particular, help to avoid the onset of the complications of massive blood transfusion.

### Retrograde urethrography

This examination is primarily for the evaluation of urethral injuries and is covered in more detail on p. 177.

### Ultrasonography

This is extremely useful in the detection of intraperitoneal fluid located in the pouch of Douglas in the female or rectovesical pouch in the male. In the setting of trauma it can quickly demonstrate major intraperitoneal haemorrhage that might be contributing to a patient's hypotension.

## Complications

### Vascular injury

The major vascular structures of the pelvis are the common, internal, and external iliac arteries, together with branches of the internal iliac arteries and their accompanying venous drainage. There is also a rich anastomotic network of vessels, both venous and arterial, throughout the entire pelvis. The paths of some of these vessels and their branches run very close to the pelvic bones and they may be injured when there is bony displacement of the fracture. Bleeding from veins is usually controlled by the tamponade effect of a closed haematoma and is usually slower than an active arterial bleed.

Fractures that are associated with significant haemorrhage include vertical shear injuries and mixed-pattern injuries. The radiological classification of pelvic fractures can provide an indication of the likelihood of significant vascular injury. However, angiography is the only means of providing a detailed assessment.

Bleeding may be massive and the retroperitoneum may hold as much as 4 litres of blood if the peritoneum remains intact. Blood transfusion is required in approximately 40 per cent of all patients with pelvic fractures, but those with unstable fractures, such as double breaks in the pelvic ring, are two and a half times more likely to require transfusion than those with stable injuries.

Anterior injuries associated with diastasis of the pubic symphysis with fracture of the pubic rami are likely to damage the pudendal, vesical, and obturator branches of the internal iliac arteries. Posterior fractures of the ilium that extend to the iliac notch may lead to damage of the superior gluteal artery, which is the largest branch of the internal iliac artery. The majority of major haemorrhages occur as a result of bleeding from the superior gluteal artery or the anterior branches of the internal iliac artery.

Fortunately these can be treated effective by a variety of embolization techniques. Early external fixation and other forms of immobilization can reduce the amount of blood loss associated with pelvic fractures. Surgical exploration to control bleeding is usually unsuccessful because of the great difficulty in identifying the bleeding vessels in the presence of haematoma. In addition, the surgical procedure may remove the tamponade effect and thus worsen the bleed. The exception is when bleeding from the large vessels can be demonstrated and when these may be accessible to surgical ligation.

## Genitourinary injury

The ureters, bladder, and urethra are found in close proximity to the bony pelvis. Failure to recognize such injuries may lead to considerable morbidity and potential mortality. The ureters are retroperitoneal in location but despite this protection are prone to injuries when fractures occur in the posterior part of the pelvis or in disruption of the sacroiliac joint. The bladder and urethra are susceptible to injury when trauma occurs anteriorly in the pelvis involving diastasis of the symphysis or fracture of the pubic rami. Urethral injuries occur almost exclusively in males, which can easily be explained by the differences in anatomy.

Clinically, gross haematuria is the most obvious sign of urinary-tract injury but may not always be present and does not correlate with the severity of injury. Clinical evaluation by means of a rectal examination may be performed to assess the prostate location. If the urethra is severed, the prostate is not felt and instead a soft boggy mass is palpable. This is often termed a 'high-riding prostate'. Should the clinical examination be inconclusive, a complete evaluation will include a retrograde urethrogram.

In cases of suspected bladder injury, such as perforation, a cystogram may be performed with the bladder distended with at least 300–400 ml of contrast, and if possible a post-drainage view is also obtained. Sometimes the leak can only be detected in the post-drainage view when the bladder mass is reduced.

## Neurological injury

The nerves that are most susceptible to injury are part of the lumbosacral plexus, and damage may occur as a result of disruption of the posterior pelvis or fractures of the sacrum, and even from posterior dislocation of the hip (avulsion of the sciatic nerve roots). The reported incidence of neurological deficits in association with pelvic fractures is approximately 12 per cent.

### Bowel injury

This is a rare complication of pelvic fracture and if present often carries a high risk of mortality. After the rectum, the small bowel is most commonly affected, especially in association with acetabular fractures. The diagnosis is often delayed because of the common occurrence of prolonged paralytic ileus in pelvic fractures. Bowel entrapment is difficult to identify on plain film in this situation but can frequently be detected by CT.

## Conclusion

With a severe pelvic injury, shock from haemorrhage or visceral injury often occur. Patients should always be stabilized before radiographic examination is performed.

Radiographic findings govern the treatment plan in most patients with pelvic injuries. Stable fractures such as single fractures are often treated conservatively. In unstable fractures, external stabilization may be required.

## BIBLIOGRAPHY

Ballinger PW. Merrill's Atlas of Radiographic Positions and Radiologic Procedures, 8th edn. Missouri: Mosby, 1995; 1:271–310.

Bulcholz RW. Pathomechanics of pelvic ring disruptions. Adv Orthop Surg 1987; 167–9.

Burgess AR, Eastridge BJ, Young JWR, *et al.* Pelvic ring disruptions; effective classification system and treatment protocols. J Trauma 1990; 30:1–9.

Cryer HM, Miller FB, Evers BM, *et al.* Pelvic fracture classification: correlation with haemorhage. J Trauma 1988; 28:973–80.

Dalal SA, Burgess AR, Siegel JH, *et al.* Pelvic fracture in multiple trauma: Classification by mechanism is key to pattern of organ injury, resuscitative requirements and outcome. J Trauma 1989; 19:981–1002.

Ellis H. Clinical Anatomy, 8th edn. Oxford; Blackwell Scientific Publications, 1992.

Epstein HC. Traumatic Dislocation of the Hip. Baltimore: Williams & Wilkins, 1980.

Helms CA. Fundamentals of Skeletal Radiology. Philadelphia: WB Saunders 1989.

Kane WJ. Fractures of the pelvis. In: Rockwood CCA, Green DP, eds. Fractures. Philadelphia: JB Lippincott, 1984; 1093–209.

Keats T. Radiology of Muscular Skeletal Stress Injury. Chicago: Year Book Medical Publishers, 1990.

Letournel E, Judet R. Fractures of the Acetabulum. Berlin: Springer-Verlag, 1981.

McCort JJ. Trauma Radiology. New York: Churchchill Livingstone, 1990.

Mack LA, Harley JD, Winquist RA. CT of acetabular fractures: analysis of fracture patterns. AJR 1982; 138:407–12.

Meschan IA. An Atlas of Anatomy Basic to Radiology. Philadelphia: WB Saunders, 1975; 2.

Pennal GF, Tile M, Wadell JP, Garside H. Pelvic disruption: asssessment and classification. Clin Orthop 1980; 151:12–21.

Rockwood CA Jr, Green DP, Bucholz RW. Rockwood and Green's Fractures in Adults, 3rd edn. Philadelphia : JB Lippincott, 1991.

Rockwood CA Jr, Wilkins KE, King RE. Fractures in Children, 3rd edn. Philadelphia: JB Lippincott, 1991; 3:754.

Tile M. Fractures of the Pelvis and Acetabulum. Baltimore: Williams & Wilkins, 1986.

Weissmann BN, Slodge CB. Orthopaedic Radiology. Philadelphia: WB Saunders, 1986.

Young JW, Burgess AR. Radiologic Management of Pelvic Ring Fractures: Systematic Radiographic Diagnosis. Baltimore: Urban and Schwarzenberg, 1987.

Young JWR, Burgess AR, Brumbach RJ, Poka A. Pelvic fractures: value of plain radiography in early assessment and management. Radiology 1986; 160:445–51.

# CHAPTER 15

# The thoracic and lumbar/sacral spine

.......................................................................................................................................................................................

- Key points: thoracic and lumbar spine

- Clinical anatomy

- Occurrence of thoracic- and lumbar-spine injuries

- The techniques available

- Imaging of specific conditions

- Bibliography

---

**Key points: thoracic and lumbar spine**

1. Conventional radiography is the initial imaging modality of choice for spinal injuries. Movement of the whole spine can be avoided by proper immobilization, and if turning is needed, the patient must be log rolled in a co-ordinated manner.

2. The views of the spine on plain radiographs, in particular of the thoracic spine, may be obscured by the overlying ribs, soft-tissue shadows, or even medical devices. CT is a useful complementary imaging modality, and subtle fractures and subluxations/dislocations are often better appreciated with this technique.

3. In the elderly population, wedged compression fractures are common, and when the loss of height of the vertebral body is greater than 50 per cent, spinal instability should be presumed.

4. The mechanism of injury will provide clues to the presence of associated fractures. For example, a fracture of the thoracolumbar spine may be associated with a calcaneal fracture in a patient who has fallen from a height onto the feet.

5. The early identification of compromise to the spinal canal and associated spinal-cord injury is essential for the early application of appropriate treatment to ensure the best neurological outcome.

# CLINICAL ANATOMY

The 12 thoracic vertebrae increase slightly in size caudally and have similar features. The five lumbar vertebrae are larger than the thoracic vertebrae and provide most of the weight-bearing function. Occasionally, sacralization of the fifth lumbar vertebra is seen when it becomes fused with the sacrum, and the first sacral vertebra may be 'lumbarized', resulting in a sixth lumbar vertebra. These are normal variants. The sacral and coccygeal vertebrae are fused together and form the posterior portion of the pelvis.

# OCCURRENCE OF THORACIC- AND LUMBAR-SPINE INJURIES

The majority of fractures and dislocations of the thoracic and lumbar spine often occur from traffic accidents, falls from a height, and certain sports. In adults, the highest frequency of fractures occurs in the region between the T11 and L4 vertebrae, and the distribution of spinal fractures commonly encountered suggests that it is important to include the lower thoracic vertebrae in the radiographic examination of lumbar-spine trauma. In children, on the other hand, fractures occur more frequently in the midthoracic and upper lumbar spine. In the elderly, wedge fractures in osteoporotic vertebral bodies are common and may result from minimal trauma.

About 10–14 per cent of spinal fractures and dislocations are associated with neurological deficit, and 20 per cent with other skeletal injuries. Some authors have reported the incidence of injury to other organs to be as high as 50 per cent.

# THE TECHNIQUES AVAILABLE

## Conventional radiography

Plain film examination is often the initial investigation of choice for suspected spinal injuries. The views obtained depend partly on the presenting clinical symptoms and signs. In addition, it should be realized that the radiograph obtained reflects the final outcome of the injury, and bony displacement may have been worse at the time of injury. Therefore, the radiographs may reveal only minimal deformities, although the total injury may be severe. The mechanism of the injury may lead to the suspicion that a more severe injury may have been sustained than that seen on the radiograph.

It is inevitable that the injured patient will be moved, whether from the accident scene to hospital, or from the A&E department to the radiology department. There is little excuse for aggravating the condition of the patient by unsafe handling, and trauma protocols that aim at spinal protection must be adhered to until full evaluation has been accomplished.

The anteroposterior (A-P) and lateral views are the routine radiographic views taken for thoracic (Fig. 15.1) and lumbar (Fig. 15.2) spine injuries. In unstable patients, a cross-table lateral view may be obtained so as to avoid further injury from patient movement. In the thoracic region the upper vertebrae are difficult to visualize satisfactorily on the lateral radiograph. A swimmer's view may be obtained instead.

In cases when the routine radiographs are apparently normal but there is a high clinical suspicion of spinal injury, CT is the investigation of choice rather than oblique views (Fig. 15.3) of the region involved, which are rarely useful. In about 10 per cent of cases where a traumatic cord injury is present there may be no overt radiographic evidence of vertebral injury. This often occurs in older patients with degenerative changes of the spine where osteophytes damage the cord, usually causing a partial cord syndrome.

Some general principles can be used in the assessment of the spine radiographs, including evaluation of the following:

1. Alignment and anatomy: the anterior and posterior margins of the vertebral bodies should be aligned to within 1 mm. The presence of large osteophytes may create difficulty in the assessment of the alignment.

2. Bony integrity: assess the shape of the bones.

3. Cartilage and joint spaces.

4. Soft-tissue abnormalities: widening of the paraspinous line in the thorax is often suggestive of a paravertebral haematoma. Apical capping on the chest radiograph is occasionally seen with fracture of the thoracic spine. The loss of the psoas margins in the lumbar film may indicate retroperitoneal haematoma as a result of a fracture of the lumbar spine. When evaluating the spine, the ribs, lungs, and mediastinum should also be assessed.

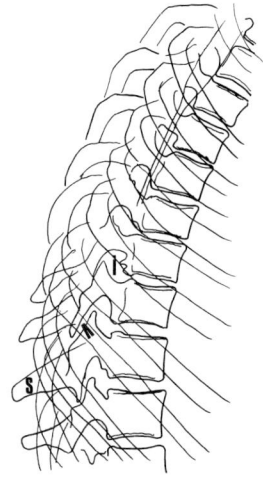

**Fig. 15.1** Thoracic spine, lateral view: I, intervertebral foramen; <, interfacet joint; s, spinous process.

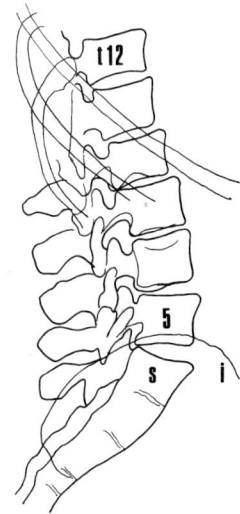

**Fig. 15.2** Lumbosacral spine, lateral view: t12, twelfth thoracic vertebral body; 5, fifth lumbar vertebral body; i, iliac crest; s, sacrum.

## Computed tomography

Although plain radiographs are still valuable as a screening tool and often serve as a guide to selective CT imaging, CT is superior to conventional radiographs in many respects.

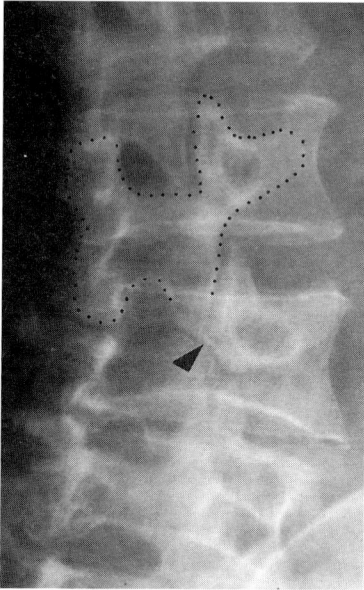

**Fig. 15.3** Lumbar spine, oblique view: . . . , normal pars interarticularis—'Scottie dog' without a collar; ◄, fractured pars interarticularis—'Scottie dog' with a collar.

There are several pitfalls in performing CT. Spines with angular deformities such as scoliosis and kyphosis may show pseudofractures on the axial images. A plain radiograph correlation can avoid diagnostic errors being made.

The present generation of CT can provide detailed anatomical information on the spine in a relatively short time period. Of particular interest is the integrity of the spinal canal, and CT can often detect subtle fractures or subluxation of the posterior aspect of the vertebrae, including the articular pillars that are difficult to visualize on plain radiographs. Often the contents of the chest and abdomen are also visualized when the corresponding thoracic and lumbar spine are scanned. This provides additional valuable information regarding associated injuries that may not be evident during the primary and secondary surveys or on initial investigation.

Routinely, axial CT images are obtained, but without sagittal or coronal reconstruction of the axial images, axially orientated fractures may be missed.

An intrathecal contrast CT myelogram may be performed to improve the evaluation of the spinal canal, and this modality has reduced the need for traditional conventional myelography that requires manipulation of the patient and therefore carries a definite risk. In hospitals with MRI facilities, intrathecal contrast CT myelogram is less frequently used, but early MRI of the injured spine of a multiple trauma victim may be impractical.

## Magnetic resonance imaging

In terms of potential benefit, MRI is the imaging modality of choice in the evaluation of the spinal cord, nerve roots, cerebrospinal fluid, intervertebral discs, ligaments, and adjacent soft tissues. Unlike CT myelography, MRI needs no contrast media to distinguish the spinal cord from the spinal fluid and surrounding soft tissue. Magnetic resonance images can be obtained in any plane without the necessity for reconstruction from the axial images or repositioning of the patient, as in CT.

In addition, post-traumatic spinal-cord atrophy and development of syringomyelia can be demonstrated well with MRI.

The presence of metallic foreign bodies, metallic prosthesis, metallic aneurysm clips, and pacemakers are known contraindications to MRI evaluation, and life-support equipment and monitors may not be compatible with MRI. In view of these limitations and the relatively poor resolution of the of bony component of the spine when compared to CT, MRI currently plays a complementary rather than alternative role to CT.

# IMAGING OF SPECIFIC CONDITIONS

## Classification of fractures

Over the years several classifications have been proposed, but none has been universally accepted. Nevertheless, classification based on the mechanism of injury appears to be more useful and allows a practical approach to these fractures. The mechanism of injury often produces a fairly predictable radiographic pattern. There are four basic mechanisms of injury which include flexion, extension, rotation, and shearing, which may occur in isolation or in combination.

Understanding the mechanism of injury allows the prediction of the possible types and stability of the fractures. Some general points include:

1. Displacement of a vertebral body suggests ligamentous disruption, which is associated with varying degrees of instability.

2. Wedge compression fractures of vertebral bodies that have caused loss of anterior height of more than 50 per cent (Fig. 15.4) are often regarded as unstable.

3. Multiple vertebral bodies with wedge compression fractures, with individual loss of anterior height of less than 50 per cent can potentially be mechanically unstable.

### Flexion injuries

Flexion injuries are by far the most common type of injury and occur as a result of a forward rotation of one vertebra over another at single or multiple levels.

### Extension injuries

Extension injuries involve primarily the cervical spine (whiplash injury) and rarely occur elsewhere in the spine. They may result in rupture of the anterior longitudinal ligament and widening of the anterior disc space, but this may not be evident on the radiograph at rest.

### Rotation injuries

Rotation injuries result from a twist of the upper body while the lower body is fixed or vice versa, often with an associated flexion component.

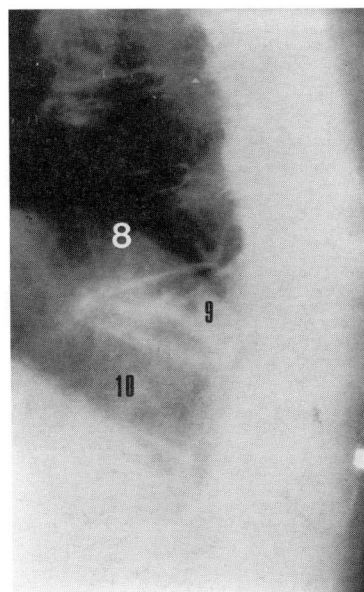

**Fig. 15.4** Thoracolumbar spine, lateral view. Wedged compression fracture of greater than 50 per cent of the anterior vertebral body vertical height: 8, eighth thoracic vertebral body; 9, ninth thoracic vertebral body with greater than 50 per cent loss of vertical height; 10, tenth thoracic vertebral body.

### Shearing injuries

Shearing injuries result from a horizontal forces acting between fixed and mobile areas of the spine, sometimes with lateral flexion. The most common situation in which this occurs is the shearing of the lumbar spine in a patient wearing a lap-only seat belt during a high-energy deceleration in a road traffic accident. These mechanisms often cause axially oriented fractures of the articular pillars with possible dislocation.

## Anterior compression fractures

This type of fracture accounts for about 48 per cent of thoracic and lumbar spine fractures. They usually result from a combination of truncal flexion and axial compression.

The lateral radiograph best demonstrates this type of fracture, showing anterior wedging or depression of the superior end plate of the vertebral body. Often there is less than 50 per cent loss of height of the anterior vertebral body (Fig. 15.5), while the height of the posterior vertebral body is preserved. The posterior structural elements are normally not affected and the spinal canal is preserved.

CT reveals comminution of the vertebral body end plate with fragments displaced in an arc-like fashion, while the posterior cortex remains intact and undisplaced. Although CT is often not required to confirm this type of fracture, occasionally when the wedge deformity is severe, or when there is accompanying neurological deficit, CT is performed to identify possible flexion–distraction or burst fracture.

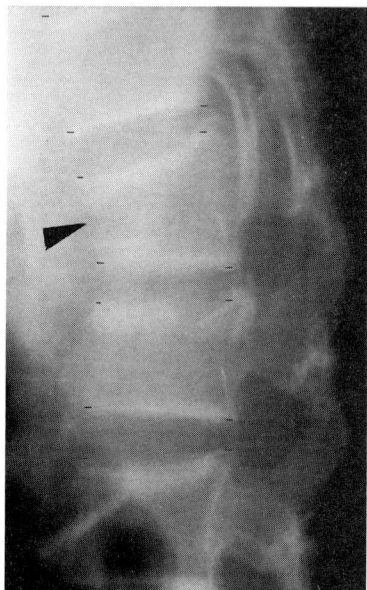

**Fig. 15.5** Thoracolumbar spine, lateral view: ►, wedged compression fracture of the first lumbar vertebral body of less than 50 per cent of the anterior vertical height (stable fracture).

## Burst fractures

Burst fractures (Fig. 15.6) result from excessive axial compression loading. Unlike the simple anterior wedge compression fractures, in burst fractures there is backward displacement of at least one fragment, arising from the posterior superior margin of the vertebral body between the pedicles, into the spinal canal. The majority of burst fractures occur at the thoracolumbar junction, with 50 per cent occurring at L1 vertebra.

About 65 per cent of patients with burst fractures will have some neurological deficit. In general, the degree of neurological injury parallels the extent of protrusion of the fracture fragments into the spinal canal.

Both anteroposterior and lateral radiographs of the spine can identify this type of fracture. On the anteroposterior view, 80 per cent of

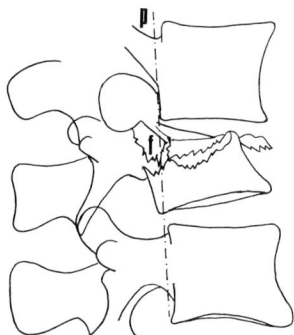

**Fig. 15.6** Lumbar spine, lateral view, burst fracture: p, disruption of the posterior bodies; f, posterior angulation and displacement of fracture fragment.

burst fractures have widening of the interpediculate distance of the fractured vertebra by 4 mm or greater when compared to the vertebra above or below the level of injury.

The radiographic indicators of instability of a burst fracture include:

(1) loss of height of the vertebral body greater than 50 per cent;

(2) increased interpediculate distance;

(3) any fracture of the pedicles, articular processes, laminae, and spinous processes.

Since fracture fragments within the spinal canal and associated fractures of the pedicles, articular processes, and laminae may be missed completely on the plain radiographs, CT is mandatory in these fractures to confirm and characterize the posterior fragment and fractured posterior elements.

If there is significant neurological deficit, MRI is valuable in assessing the spinal cord and nerve roots at the site of abnormality, usually at a later stage.

## Flexion–distraction injuries

This type of injury results from a greater degree of compression force that increases the likelihood of the presence of posterior element fractures (pedicles, articular processes, and laminae). The radiographs may demonstrate absence or minimal anterior body compression with any of the following features:

(1) widening of the interspinous distance;

(2) separation of the spinous processes;

(3) a distracted fracture of the spinous process;

(4) dissociation of the articular processes;

(5) widening of the disc space.

## Facet subluxation/dislocation

Bilateral or unilateral facet dislocation of the thoracolumbar spine is rare. The mechanism of injury is hyperflexion without axial loading or flexion–rotation without axial loading, respectively. These are often associated with ligamentous injury, which gives rise to potential spinal instability. Occasionally, fracture of the facet occurs due to the shearing forces.

## Fracture–dislocation (translation) injuries

This type of injury is the result of a combination of flexion, axial compression, and rotational shearing forces. When these occur in the upper eight thoracic vertebrae and thoracolumbar junction, neurological deficits are often encountered. These fractures rarely occur at the lumbosacral junction.

The radiological features may include anterior displacement of the spine above the injury, accompanied by a variable degree of anterior wedging of the vertebra below, often with a characteristic triangular fragment sheared from the anterior superior margin. In addition, tears of the supraspinous and infraspinous ligaments and disruption of the facets, with accompanying fractures of the superior facets and laminae, are often found.

Simply placing the patient's shoulders in line with the pelvis may partially reduce this fracture dislocation, and therefore radiographs taken after the injury may demonstrate less displacement than that which occurred during the injury.

It may be difficult to visualize these injuries on plain radiographs of the upper thoracic spine. However, the presence of a pleural cap resulting from haematoma dissecting over the apex of the lung, or misalignment of the spinous processes, are indirect signs that should raise suspicion.

## Fractures of the transverse processes

These fractures may result from sudden forceful contractions of the paraspinal muscles or occasionally from direct blows. The fractures are orientated vertically or obliquely and the vertebral bodies are otherwise intact.

If the fracture line is orientated horizontally, care should be taken to exclude the presence of a Chance fracture. Avulsion fractures of the fifth lumbar transverse process are often associated with pelvic disruption. This is due the presence of the iliolumbar ligament that connects the transverse process to the ilium.

## Chance fracture/seat-belt fracture

With the introduction of seat-belt laws, there has been a well-documented reduction in motor vehicle accident mortality and morbidity. However, this has resulted in the appearance of a special type of hyperflexion injury.

The common hyperflexion injury of the spine occurs with the fulcrum in the posterior portion of the vertebral body, leading to a wedge compression fracture. With seat-belt fractures, the fulcrum is brought forward to the seat belt, which results in an unusual lumbar fracture.

On the anteroposterior film, fractures of the posterior elements may be recognized. Usually there is a horizontal lucency across the pedicle, breaking its cortical continuity. Occasionally the fracture may extend anteriorly into the posterior part of the vertebral body. Compression fracture of the vertebral body is often minimal. Lateral radiographs of the lumbar spine can be obtained for confirmation.

This fracture, when imaged on CT in the axial plane, may be difficult to appreciate. The sagittal- and coronal-plane reformatted images are often required to fully define the injury.

Injuries to the spinal cord and cauda equina may accompany this fracture. In addition, intra-abdominal injuries to the duodenum, small bowel, spleen, and pancreas may occur secondary to visceral compression by the seat belt.

## Multiple-level spinal injuries

These occur in about 4 per cent of all patients with spinal injuries and are seen more often in patients with accompanying neurological deficit. Therefore patients who have sustained a cord injury should be assessed carefully for additional fractures, ideally with a thorough CT examination.

# BIBLIOGRAPHY

Angtuaco EJC, Binet EF. Radiology of thoracic and lumbar fractures. Clin Orthop 1984; 189:43–57.

Ballinger PW. Merrill's Atlas of Radiographic Positions and Radiologic Procedures, 8th edn. Missouri: Mosby, 1995; 1:324–98.

Daffner RH. Imaging of Vertebra Trauma. Rockville, MD: Aspen Publishers, 1988.

Daffner RH, Deeb ZL, Rothfus WE. 'Fingerprints' of vertebral trauma—a unifying concept based on mechanisms. Skeletal Radiol 1986; 15:518–25.

Errico JT, Bauer RD, Waugh T. Spinal Trauma. Philadelphia: JB Lippincott, 1991.

Hollinshead WH, Rosse C. Textbook of Anatomy, 4th edn. Philadelphia: Harper and Row, 1985.

Keats TE. Atlas of Normal Roentgen Variants that may Simulate Disease, 5th edn. St Louis: Mosby Year Book, 1992.

Meschan IA. An Atlas of Anatomy Basic to Radiology. Philadelphia: WB Saunders, 1975.

Resnick D. Bone and Joint Imaging. Philadelphia: WB Saunders, 1989.

Rockwood CA Jr, Green DP, Bucholz RW. Rockwood and Green's Fractures in Adults, 3rd edn. Philadelphia: JB Lippincott, 1991.

Rogers LF. Radiology of Skeletal Trauma. New York: Churchill Livingstone, 1982.

# CHAPTER 16

# *The extremities*

- Key points: the extremities
- Clinical assessment
- Upper limb
- Lower limb
- Paediatric injuries
- Bibliography

---

### Key points: the extremities

1. Joint dislocations associated with vascular or skin compromise should be reduced promptly. Often this is necessary even before radiographic confirmation of the injury, relying instead on diagnostic clinical features.

2. In multiple trauma victims, skin folds, bandages, medical devices, or other overlying materials may simulate fracture lines on the plain radiographs. Clinical correlation is required to exclude these artefacts.

3. Long-bone fractures may be associated with significant blood loss, but the radiographic appearances seldom show this directly. The presence of comminution may indicate fractures which are prone to major blood loss.

4. In children, the unfused apophyses or ossification centres should not be mistaken for fractures.

---

## CLINICAL ASSESSMENT

Bony injuries of the extremities are common and form the 'bread and butter' of trauma work in the A&E department. In the majority of cases the patterns of injuries can be recognized from the type of mechanism of injury. The majority of musculoskeletal injuries are not life threatening but major joint dislocations, amputation, open fractures, and the development of compartment syndromes may result in the loss of an extremity. Limb injuries may be missed in the multiple trauma patient, due to the presence of more spectacular or urgent problems.

Plain radiographic evaluation of the extremities in trauma is the mainstay of the diagnosis of fractures in the A&E department. In addition, both radiopaque and radiolucent foreign bodies can be detected with these simple investigations. Radiolucent foreign bodies may be difficult to detect but the presence of indirect radiological signs and clinical examination can help.

Often the site of maximum tenderness suggests a possible fracture of the underlying bone. History taking and clinical examination assist in ensuring that the appropriate radiographic views are obtained. Plain radiographs assist in detecting or confirming the presence of a fracture and also allow evaluation of their severity. In addition, plain radiographs may identify the presence of an underlying bone disease such as osteoporosis.

As with the evaluation of other bones, routine examination usually consists of two perpendicular views including the anteroposterior and lateral projections. Occasionally, oblique views may be needed to demonstrate a fracture. When permitted, the film should include the entire bone as well as the joints above and below it.

In multiple trauma victims, skin folds, bandages, or other overlying material such as linen may simulate fracture lines, and the clinician may have to repeat a careful clinical examination to exclude these artefacts if unexpected appearances are found on the radiographs.

Even with the best of radiographic techniques, some fractures (such as fracture of the scaphoid) may not demonstrate a fracture line initially. On a repeat radiograph 7–10 days after the injury, the margins of the fracture are often absorbed and widening of the fracture or radiolucent line occurs, making the previously undetected fracture obvious. Also, follow-up examinations are often warranted if pain persists, even though initial radiographs of the limb were normal.

On occasion, stress views are used to evaluate the extent of ligamentous injuries. Stress manoeuvres should be performed only under the direction of the ordering physician. Stress views are generally contraindicated in young patients with suspected epiphyseal injury or fracture. In some situations, any applied stress may worsen the injury.

It pays to be meticulous in examining the entire radiograph right up to the film edge, and not to be overwhelmed by the discovery of the first fracture, because the most commonly missed fractures are second fractures on the same film.

Elaborate classifications of fractures are not always useful early in the management of patients with multiple trauma, as they are often complicated and it is more important to establish priorities in management. However, if a fracture is present, it should be simply categorized when possible. The fracture is frequently termed open or closed, depending on whether the fracture communicates with the outside environment (this includes gut and sinuses). It is common to have open fractures in multiple trauma victims, reflecting the high energy transfer involved or the presence of penetrating injuries. With open fractures, foreign materials within the fracture site should be carefully excluded on clinical and radiological examination.

Single fracture lines are often described as transverse or spiral. A transverse fracture usually indicates injury caused by significant local force, while a spiral fracture would imply a twisting injury. When there is more than a single fracture line, the fracture is termed comminuted.

The orientation of the distal fragment with respect to the proximal bone assists further in description, including whether the bone is angulated, rotated, or displaced.

Description of intra-articular extension, associated subluxations or dislocations, and soft-tissue foreign bodies may assist in planning management.

Pathological fractures may occur through an already abnormal bone. In most instances, these fractures occur with a smaller amount of force than would be required to injure a normal bone.

CT may be useful in evaluating complex fractures, when the limbs are in a cast or heavy dressing. The added advantage of multiplanar image reformatting and imaging in three dimensions has increased the usefulness of CT in the evaluation of both major and minor trauma. Complex articular surface fractures are well defined by two- or three-dimensional reformatting, allowing better appreciation of the injury than with transaxial imaging alone. The fracture line may be missed when it parallels the transaxial plane of a CT image. Artefacts from metallic surgical implants or bullet fragments can occur with CT, but these can be reduced by reformatting.

MRI of musculoskeletal injuries can produce images in virtually any plane desired and, coupled with excellent soft-tissue contrast resolution, this imaging modality is ideal for identifying injuries to all structures. However, long scanning time, constraints in evaluating cortical bone, the presence of ferromagnetic foreign bodies, or life-support equipment that is not suitable for use with MRI, all limit the use of MRI in the emergency setting.

Scintigraphy is not frequently used in the emergency department, but in some situations bone radionuclide scans are helpful. These include the detection of occult scaphoid and femoral neck fractures and evaluation of the physically abused child.

Complications of fractures include those with immediate and those with long-term sequelae. Immediate complications commonly involve soft-tissue damage, including compartment syndrome which, left unchecked, can lead to progressive ischaemia and ultimate necrosis of muscle and a threat to the limb. Sometimes the threat can be anticipated from the severity of the radiographic findings.

Arterial injuries may occur as a result of laceration by sharp bony fragments, from a penetrating injury, or from avulsion or traction injuries. The absence of distal pulses would suggest a possible arterial injury. Frequently, angiography is required to evaluate the extent and location of such injuries.

Long-term sequelae of fractures include avascular necrosis, non-union, deformities such as limb shortening, infection, and post-traumatic ossification, and arthritis. All of these can be assessed with the imaging techniques described.

# UPPER LIMB

## Clavicle

Fractures of the clavicle are relatively common and often occur as isolated injuries, usually resulting from a fall on the outstretched hand or directly onto the shoulder. Clavicular fractures occur in the middle third in approximately 80 per cent of cases, in the outer third in 15 per cent, and in the medial third in 5 per cent of cases.

The routine radiographic view of the clavicle consists of a straight anteroposterior projection with a slight rostral angulation to project the clavicles off the ribs. In the majority of cases, fractures of the middle third can be seen with this view. The fracture is made obvious as the medial fragment is usually displaced upwards by the pull of the sternocleidomastoid muscle, while the lateral fragment is pulled downwards by the pectoralis minor muscle and the weight of the arm. However, when there is little or no displacement of the fracture components, an angled anteroposterior or oblique view may be required to demonstrate the fracture adequately.

Occasionally, fractures of the middle third of the clavicle can be associated with severe soft-tissue injury, in particular to the subclavian artery. Clinically this is usually accompanied by a weak or absent radial pulse.

Fractures of the sternoclavicular joint can also be difficult to detect, as underlying and neighbouring bony structures may obscure the region. These include the thoracic spine and ribs. Unfortunately, these fractures can be associated with serious injuries to the underlying mediastinal structures, including the great vessels, and may be potentially life threatening. Oblique views may show these fractures but CT of the region demonstrates the fractures best, and can also assess the underlying soft tissues.

Fractures of the outer third may involve the acromioclavicular joint and may predispose to osteoarthritis.

## Shoulder including scapula

In the majority of injuries involving the shoulder, plain radiographs will provide sufficient diagnostic information. However, in the presence of complex fractures and the need to assess underlying soft-tissue structures, computed tomography is usually required.

The shoulder girdle consists of the clavicle and scapula. These articulate with one another at the acromioclavicular joint (Fig. 16.1) and with the humerus at the glenohumeral joint, to form the shoulder joint.

The routine radiographic examination of the shoulder includes the neutral anteroposterior view. In this view the greater tuberosity is projected at the upper outer margin of the humerus. The glenoid fossa is not seen in its entirety but its margins can be made out with acceptable clarity. The acromion process articulates with the clavicle is also well visualized. In general, this view includes the distal end of the clavicle, scapula, and the proximal humerus.

Of the many special views of the shoulder, the axillary view (Fig. 16.2) is extremely useful, but may be difficult to obtain in a seriously injured patient. A slightly modified view can be obtained without the patient needing to abduct the arm 90° from the body. In the axillary view, the coracoid process is projected anteriorly with the acromion

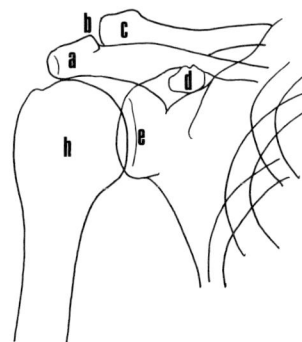

**Fig. 16.1** Shoulder, anterior view: a, acromion; b, acromioclavicular joint; c, coracoid process; e, glenoid.

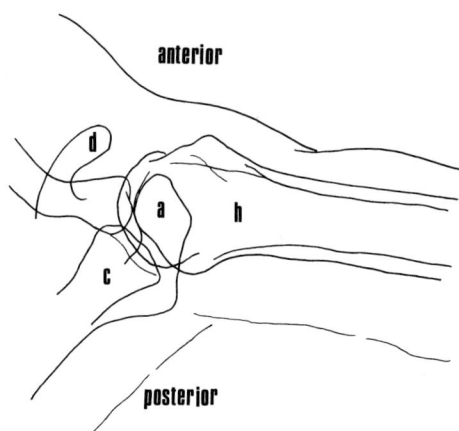

**Fig. 16.2** Shoulder, axial view: a, acromion; c, clavicle; d, coracoid process; h, humerus.

process posteriorly. The advantage is that it can provide conclusive evidence of posterior shoulder dislocation suspected on the antero-posterior view, and minimally displaced fractures of the coracoid process of the scapula.

The shoulder is the most frequently dislocated joint in the body. Although usually clinically evident, radiography is needed to deter-mine the direction of dislocation and for detection of associated frac-tures. Anterior dislocation of the shoulder is easily detected on the anteroposterior view of the shoulder (Fig. 16.3). Anterior shoulder dislocations are common and usually occur during excessive external rotation with the arm in abduction. This may be associate with Hill–Sachs fracture of the humeral head, Bankart's fracture of the inferior glenoid, and fracture of the greater tuberosity. Glenoid frac-tures associated with shoulder dislocation are frequently seen on the anteroposterior view of the shoulder. Fractures of the coracoid process may also be associated with shoulder dislocation but are difficult to detect on the anteroposterior view. If there is minimal dis-placement, an axillary view will be helpful.

The relatively uncommon posterior dislocation (Fig. 16.4) may be missed, both clinically and radiologically. The most common cause is

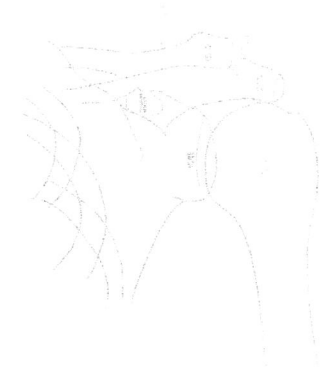

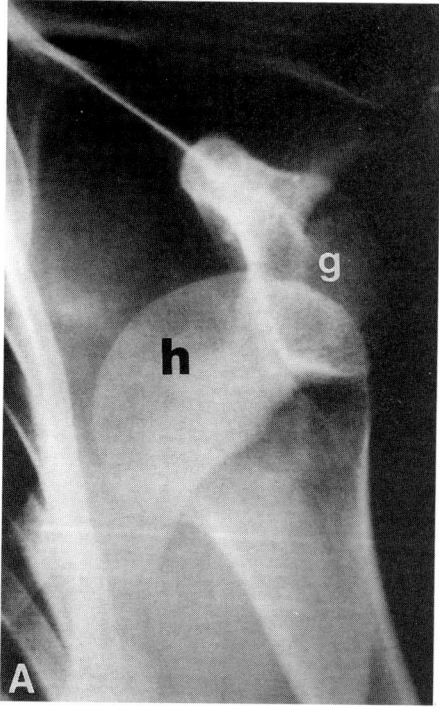

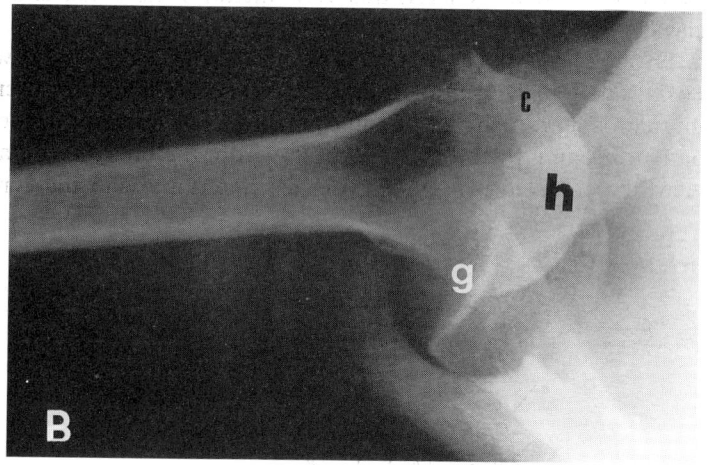

**Fig. 16.3**  Shoulder, anterior dislocation: (A) anteroposterior view; (B) axial view. c, Coracoid process; g, glenoid fossa of the scapula is not articulating with h, the head of the humerus.

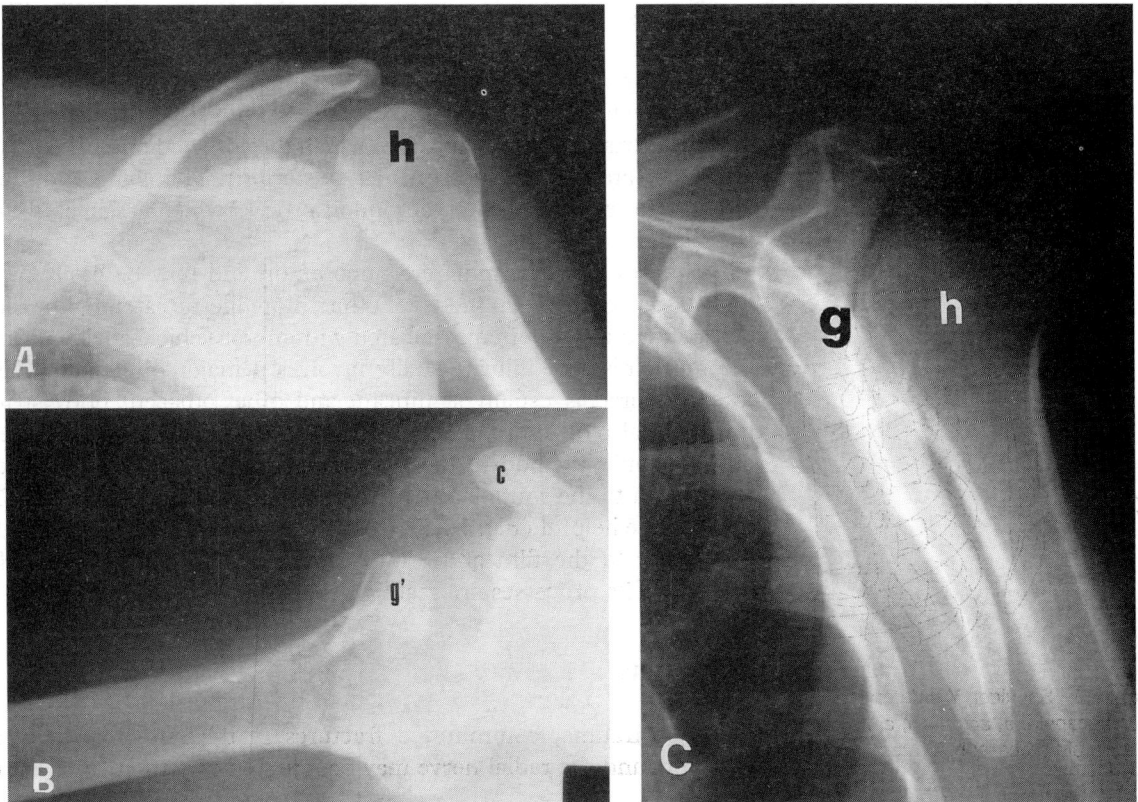

**Fig. 16.4** Shoulder, posterior dislocation. (A) Anteroposterior view, dislocated humeral head resembling a 'light bulb'. (B) Axial view; g', fracture fragment from glenoid. (C) Lateral or Y view of the scapula; g, glenoid fossa not articulating with h, the humeral head.

a tonic–clonic seizure with violent internal rotation of the humerus. On examination, patients may have difficulty in abducting the arm and have a persistent severe internal rotation of the humerus, which on the anteroposterior view of the shoulder shows the humeral head to resemble a light bulb. There may be incongruity between the humeral head and the glenoid fossa, with superimposition of the humeral head on the fossa. In equivocal cases, an axillary view can be obtained to confirm the clinical suspicion.

The acromioclavicular joint is the other joint that is commonly dislocated or subluxed. The anteroposterior view may include stress views with and without weights in both hands, to accentuate any separation. The normal acromioclavicular joint is approximately 4 mm wide but should be less than 8 mm. However, the difference between the two acromioclavicular joints in any individual should be less than 3 mm. Of importance is a complete disruption of the coracoclavicular ligament, which supports the upper limb. This

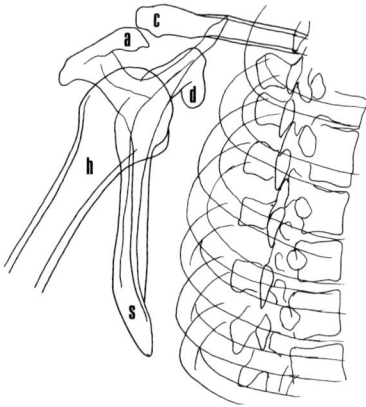

**Fig. 16.5** Shoulder, Y or lateral view of the scapula: a, acromion; c, clavicle; d, coracoid process; h, humerus; s, scapula.

may be suspected when the coracoclavicular separation is more than 1.3 cm.

The scapula is a large, flat bone on the dorsal aspect of the thorax. It normally lies between the second and seventh ribs. The body of the scapula is triangular in shape from which the coracoid process extends anteriorly and the spine protrudes posteriorly. The spine continues laterally to terminate as the acromion process which articulates with the clavicle.

Fractures of the scapula are uncommon and may be easily overlooked, especially when there are other, more life-threatening injuries. These fractures are often associated with motor vehicle accidents and the mechanism of injury usually involves a major direct blow. The force required is usually significant and other adjacent bony structures may also be injured, including the ribs and clavicles. Of the parts of the scapula, the body is the most commonly fractured. Sometimes, in addition to the routine anteroposterior view, a lateral scapular (Y) view can be helpful (Fig. 16.5). In this view the scapula is placed perpendicular to the film and any fractures in the main body of the scapula or its processes are readily detected.

## Humerus

In major trauma, comminuted fractures of the humeral shaft are common, and the radial nerve may be injured in up to 30 per cent of cases.

Fractures of the proximal and distal humerus may also involve the shoulder and the elbow joints. The brachial plexus and axillary vessels may be injured in cases of proximal humerus fracture with significant displacement.

Clinically, any angulation of the arm makes the diagnosis obvious and usually anteroposterior and lateral radiographs would be sufficient to demonstrate the severity of the fracture. On the anteroposterior view of the arm, most of the anatomical parts of the humerus are identified. These include the head, neck, greater and lesser tubercles, intertubercular groove, deltoid tubercle, both medial and lateral epicondyles, olecranon fossa, and the capitellum and trochlea, which articulate with the radius and ulna respectively. On the lateral radiograph of the arm, the medial and lateral epicondyles are projected over one another. The cubital fossa is seen in profile. The presence of associated vascular and neurological injuries will usually require surgical intervention at an early stage.

## Elbow

The elbow is a hinge joint in which the humerus articulates with the ulna and head of the radius. In addition, the head of radius articulates with the radial notch of the coronoid process of the ulna. The two portions of the joint have a direct communication.

Most elbow injuries are caused by indirect trauma transmitted through the forearm. Routine radiographic examination for the elbow includes the anteroposterior and lateral projections. Occasionally, oblique views may be required to demonstrate clinically suspected fractures. Sometimes an abnormal olecranon fat pad sign is the only obvious radiographic sign of intra-articular fractures, and is seen on a lateral view.

The lateral radiograph of the elbow requires precise positioning, especially for the evaluation of the fragments of a supracondylar fracture. Small degrees of rotation in the lateral view have been known to cause misleading results, such as the obscuring of minimally displaced or undisplaced supracondylar fractures, false positive olecranon fat pad sign, and incorrectly demonstrated alignment of the fragments.

In evaluating elbow injuries, two important lines should be determined. These are the anterior humeral line and the proximal mid-radial line (Fig. 16.6). On the lateral view, the anterior humeral line is the downward extension of the anterior cortex of the distal humeral shaft. This line intersects with the capitellum near the junction of the anterior and middle third of the capitellum. Any alteration of the line should raise the suspicion of subtle capitellar epiphyseal and transcondylar fractures. The other line, the proximal mid-radial line, is drawn from the mid-radial shaft, beginning at the level of the radial tubercle and extending proximally through the radial head, and this line normally bisects the capitellum. Any alteration in the line suggests subtle radial-head dislocation.

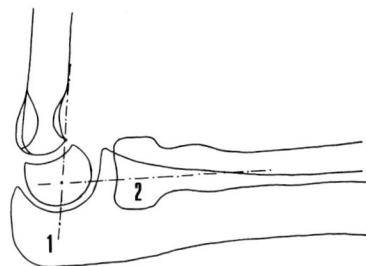

**Fig. 16.6** Elbow, lateral view: 1, anterior humeral line intersects the capitellum near the junction of the anterior and middle third of the capitellum; 2, proximal mid-radial line normally bisects the capitellum.

Evaluation of the elbow includes the elbow fat pads. The anterior fat pad is normally visualized on the anterior aspect of the elbow on the lateral radiograph but becomes more prominent or assumes a sail appearance when there is a joint effusion or haemarthrosis. The posterior fat pad in the intercondylar depression is only seen when there is an intra-articular collection. The posterior fat pad sign is usually a more sensitive indicator of joint effusion.

In adults the most common injuries of the elbow are fractures of the radial head or neck. The mechanism usually involves a fall onto the outstretched hand in supination. Occasionally, subtle fractures may not be identified in any of the views and the only radiographic sign is an elevated olecranon (posterior) fat pad sign. When present, this sign indicates the need for follow-up, possibly including a further radiograph 10–14 days later which may demonstrate any fracture more clearly.

Comminuted fractures of the distal humerus with extension into the elbow are often associated with dislocations around the elbow. However, elbow dislocation can also occur without any fractures, and any injury of significant severity to the elbow can result in vascular and neurological damage.

## Forearm

Fractures of the radius or ulna or both are also occasionally associated with dislocations of the elbow or distal radioulnar joint. The routine radiographic views of the forearm therefore include the anteroposterior and lateral views extending to both the wrist and elbow. Examples of potential injury patterns include the Monteggia fracture (ulnar fracture with radial-head dislocation) and Galeazzi fracture (radial fracture with ulnar dislocation).

Treatment of fractures of the radial and ulnar shafts may require radiological assistance. It is important that reduction of the fractures should be precise in order to restore function, and an image intensifier may be used to screen the fracture position dynamically during reduction.

## Wrist

Most injuries to the wrist result from a fall on the outstretched hand. The routine radiographic views of the wrist include anteroposterior, lateral, and both oblique views. The oblique views maximize the visibility of the scaphoid bone.

It is also equally important for the examining physician to indicate precisely the anatomical region to be radiographed, for example by requesting scaphoid views when maximum tenderness is elicited in the anatomical snuffbox, or a carpal-tunnel view when there is a suspicion of a fracture of the hook of the hamate or of the pisiform.

The anteroposterior radiograph includes the distal radius and ulna, carpal bones, and the bases of the metacarpals. The normal relationship of the carpal bones demonstrates the bones in two rows, and all the bones have about the same 2–3 mm joint space. Any widening of the spaces would indicate ligamentous disruption in the wrist.

The lateral view is valuable in the assessment of the alignment of the distal forearm fracture fragment, the radiocarpal angle, and also any carpal and carpometacarpal dislocation or subluxation. In the normal wrist in the neutral position, a straight line can be drawn through the long axis of the radius, lunate, and capitate. Angulation of this line would indicate carpal instability.

The carpus consists of eight bones arranged in two rows that articulate in a concavoconvex manner. The scaphoid, lunate, triquetral, and pisiform form the proximal row. The distal row consists of the trapezium (greater multangular), trapezoid (lesser multangular), capitate, and hamate. Short intercarpal ligaments bind the carpal bones to each other. The proximal articulation of the wrist is formed by the radius articulating with the scaphoid and lunate.

The most common fracture in the wrist involves the distal radius and ulna. Colles fracture commonly occurs as the result of a fall onto an outstretched hand, producing a fracture of the distal radius with dorsal angulation of the distal fragment. Clinically the fracture results in a 'dinner fork' deformity of the wrist. Also, there is a fracture of the ulnar styloid in up to 60 per cent of cases.

The less common Smith's fracture is the reverse of the Colles fracture and results from forced flexion of the wrist. The distal fragment of the radius demonstrates a volar angulation. Barton's or reverse Barton's fractures are similar to Colles and Smith's fractures with the addition of an intra-articular extension. In these cases there may be additional subluxation or dislocation of the carpal bones.

Subluxation or dislocation of the distal radio-ulnar joint is often difficult to identify on plain radiographs alone. These features commonly occur in association with distal radial fractures but may occur in isolation. The dislocation occurs secondary to disruption of the dorsal ligaments, with injury to the triangular fibrocartilage complex. The radio-ulnar instability is more pronounced on supination or pronation. The distal radio-ulnar joint plays an important role in integrated forearm, wrist, and hand function, and injuries can result in loss of ability to perform manual work subsequently. Therefore, in clinically suspicious cases, computed tomography should be employed to demonstrate these abnormalities and plan repair.

## Carpal injuries

The scaphoid bone is the most common carpal bone to be fractured and, around the wrist, second only to fractures of the distal radius. The initial radiographic study may fail to demonstrate any fracture but in cases with a suggestive injury mechanism, a repeat radiograph 1–2 weeks after immobilization should be obtained. In the majority of cases, any fracture line not visible earlier becomes apparent. The majority of fractures occur at the waist, and less commonly at the proximal pole. The precautionary approach to possible scaphoid fractures in clinically suspicious cases is followed because failure to identify the fracture may lead to non-union and osteonecrosis with delayed morbidity. However, this is unlikely to occur with undisplaced injuries, and failure to suspect injury and order initial radiographs is a more common reason for patients developing such avoidable complications.

Fractures of the other carpal bones are uncommon, but subluxations and dislocation occur more frequently. Fracture of the triquetrum is the second most common fracture of the carpus, and the diagnosis is easily made on a good lateral film. Clinical examination elicits pain and tenderness over the affected bone and the fracture can be located usually with significant accuracy with a review of the anatomy on the radiograph. Fractures of the hook of hamate and pisiform usually will require carpal-tunnel views to establish a radiological diagnosis.

Scapholunate dissociation is identified on the anteroposterior view from the widening of the scapholunate joint by more than 3 mm. This sign is also seen in rotational dislocation of the scaphoid.

In lunate dislocation (Fig. 16.7), the anteroposterior view shows the lunate appearing more triangular in shape as opposed to the normal rectangular shape. Also, the lunate is seen to overlap the capitate, hamate, and triquetrum. The lateral view is rather more dramatic with the lunate seen displaced from the carpus, usually on the volar aspect. A properly positioned lateral view of the wrist is essential in this case, or the dislocation may be missed.

In perilunate dislocation (which may occur with or without a fracture of the scaphoid), the carpus is dislocated posteriorly with respect to the lunate. Clinically there is associated deformity, swelling, and marked limitation of the wrist movement. Radiographs show wrist shortening and an increase in overlap of the carpal bones. Again the

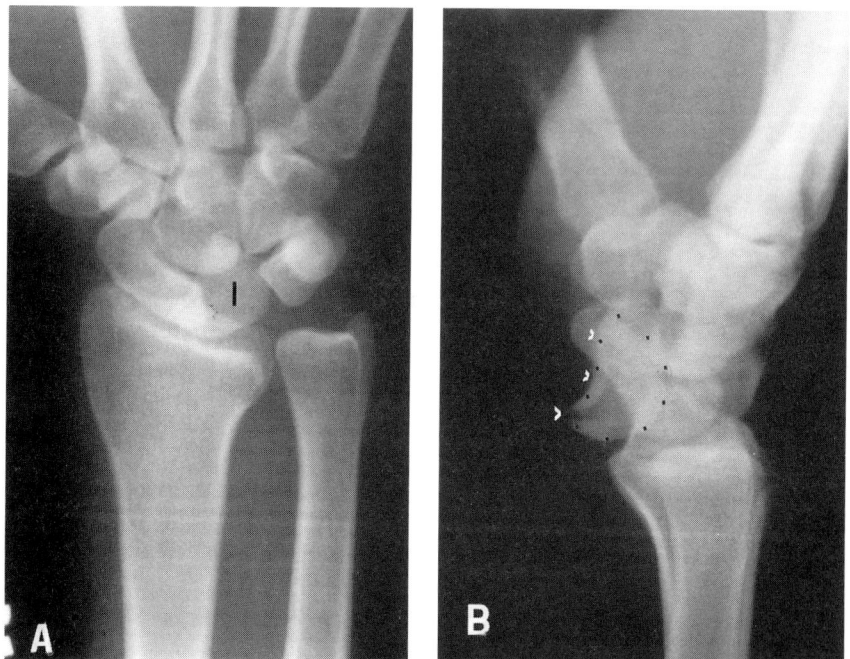

**Fig. 16.7** Wrist, lunate dislocation. (A) Frontal view; 1, lunate appears more triangular in shape and overlaps with the capitate, hamate, and triquetrum. (B) Lateral view; v, lunate—volar displacement from the carpus.

dislocation is better demonstrated on the lateral view. The lunate maintains a normal alignment with the distal radius, but there is absence of the capitate from the lunate cap, and also the rest of the carpus is seen to be dislocated posteriorly with respect to the lunate.

Dislocations of the carpometacarpal joints other than the thumb are uncommon, and if present are often associated with fracture at the base of the metacarpal or adjacent carpal bones. These cases usually result from direct trauma.

# Hand

The routine radiographic study of the hand includes posteroanterior (frontal), lateral, and occasionally oblique views.

The hand (Fig. 16.8) consists of five metacarpals, and three phalanges for each digit except for the thumb, which has two. Sesamoid bones are commonly encountered as small, rounded bones embedded in flexor tendons on the volar side of the digital rays.

## Metacarpals

The metacarpals articulate with the carpus proximally and the phalanges distally. The first metacarpal is the shortest and thickest, while the second is usually the longest. In the immature skeleton, the epiphysis of the first metacarpal is found at the base, instead of at the head as found in the rest of the metacarpals. This should not be mistaken for a fracture.

Although injuries may appear to be limited to a digit, radiographic study of the entire hand is advisable if the injury mechanism is not precisely localized, as there may be associated, clinically unsuspected fractures.

The thumb metacarpal deserves special mention because of its anatomy. An anteroposterior radiographic view of the hand will not demonstrate a frontal view of the thumb, and therefore an additional view required. More than three-quarters of fractures of the first metacarpal involve the base and half of them are intra-articular. Bennett's fracture is the most common injury of the first metacarpal and involves fracture of the proximal metacarpal with intra-articular involvement. It is liable to be unstable, and early orthopaedic management is required.

Metacarpal shaft fractures commonly occur in an oblique or spiral manner through the shaft. The most common metacarpal fracture involves the neck of the fifth (and occasionally the fourth) metacarpal, usually due to direct trauma and known as the 'boxer's fracture'. These patients have a history of striking a blow with a clenched fist.

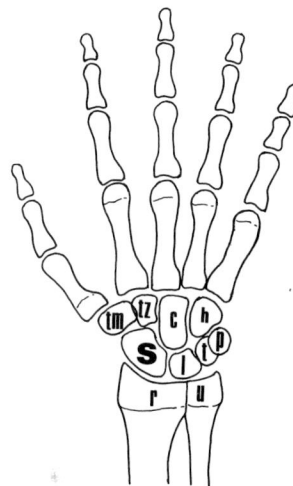

**Fig. 16.8** Hand, frontal view: tm, trapezium; tz, trapezoid; c, capitate; h, hamate; p, pisiform; t, triquetrum; l, lunate; s, scaphoid; r, radius; u, ulna.

Although fractures with angulation and rotation are easily identified, minimally displaced fractures may be difficult to recognize unless two views are taken at an angle to each other.

**Phalanges**

In the elderly, there is a tendency for the margins of the shafts in areas of muscular/tendon attachment to become increasingly more irregular, and these appearances may be confused with fractures.

Normal sesamoid bones are most frequently seen as a pair of small, rounded bones over the thumb metacarpophalangeal joint, a single one over the interphalangeal joint of the thumb, and one over the metacarpophalangeal joint of the fifth finger. These should not be mistaken for fracture fragments.

The routine radiographic views include anteroposterior and oblique views. The advantage of the oblique view over the lateral projection is that there is no significant overlap of the various anatomical regions of the hand. The straight lateral view is necessary to demonstrate the degree of anteroposterior displacement in a fracture, but is usually only taken for the specific digit that is injured, rather than the whole hand.

It is essential to remember that what appear to be radiographically trivial fractures of the phalanges may produce great functional disability. Also, in phalangeal dislocations, fractures may be more evident on the postreduction films, hence the importance of repeating the radiological examination after reduction. Lack of congruity of the joint may suggest interposition of soft tissue in the joint, and may be associated with difficulty in reduction or subsequent instability.

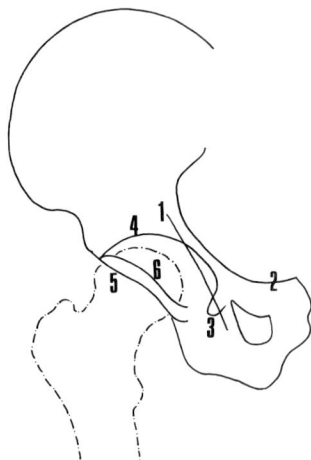

**Fig. 16.9** Hip, anteroposterior view: 1, ilioischial line; 2, iliopubic line; 3, teardrop; 4, acetabulum roof and medial wall; 5, posterior lip of acetabulum; 6, anterior lip of acetabulum.

# LOWER LIMB

## Hip

The routine radiographic views of the hip include the anteroposterior pelvis (Fig. 16.9) and lateral views of the hip (Fig. 16.10). The full anteroposterior view of the pelvis, and not a limited view of the hip, should be obtained to allow for comparison of the two sides and also for the diagnosis of pubic ramus fractures. This is most important when the patient complains of pain and the hip appears normal.

In the normal radiograph, the Shenton line is a smooth, curved line that runs from the inferior border of the femoral neck to the inferior surface of the superior pubic rami. Most fractures of the hip will disrupt this line. In taking the anteroposterior view (Fig. 16.11), the

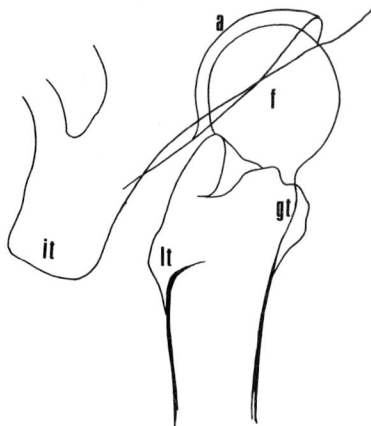

**Fig. 16.10** Hip, lateral view: a, acetabular rim; f, head of femur; gt, greater trochanter; it, ischial tuberosity; lt, lesser trochanter.

limb is best rotated internally to ensure adequate visualization of the femoral neck, otherwise the neck may appear foreshortened. To the unfamiliar, this appearance may mimic an impacted fracture, but fortunately most impacted fractures are evident by a thin sclerotic line. It is important not to miss this diagnosis, as an impacted non-displaced fracture may be converted into a displaced one by weight bearing, with subsequent complications such as avascular necrosis and non-union. The lateral view enables adequate visualization of the entire acetabulum, ischial tuberosity, and neck of femur.

The frog-leg lateral view of the hip provides an imperfect but useful view of the head, neck, and upper shaft of the femur, but the acetabulum remains demonstrated in the anteroposterior relationship. This view is commonly used for suspected abnormalities in children when the acetabulum lateral view is not necessary. This view is contraindicated if a fracture is suspected, when hip motion is extremely limited and painful.

In obese patients, overlying skin folds may mimic fractures. Fortunately this is not a common problem as most skin-fold markings extend beyond the bone into the soft tissue.

Dislocation of the hip is commonly due to axial forces transmitted along the femoral shaft during abrupt deceleration, such as in a motor vehicle accident. This results in a posterior dislocation with some superior displacement of the femoral head. However, when the thigh is forcibly abducted during the impact (particularly common in motorcycle accidents), there may be an associated fracture of the posterior acetabular lip. In many cases, the patella may also be fractured. Anterior dislocation of the hip does occur but much less frequently, the majority being secondary to motor vehicle accidents but occasionally resulting from a fall or a blow to the back while squatting. In these cases, there may be associated impacted fracture of the femoral head, caused when it hits the anterior acetabular rim.

CT is usually required to identify osteochondral fractures or fragments, which may be the reason why a dislocated hip proves resistant to reduction. Complications of hip dislocation include failed reduction, recurrent dislocation, avascular necrosis of femoral head (especially when the dislocation is not reduced within the first few hours), osteoarthritis, myositis ossificans, sciatic nerve and femoral nerve palsy, and arterial compression in anterior dislocation.

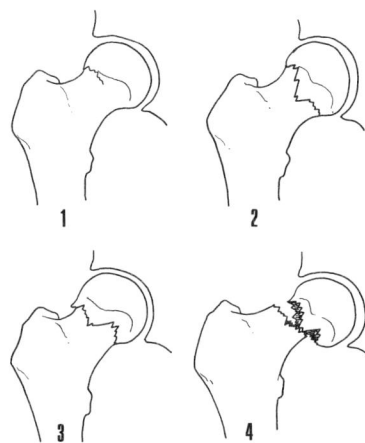

**Fig. 16.11** Hip, anteroposterior view, fractured neck of femur: 1, incomplete fracture; 2, complete fracture without displacement; 3, complete fracture with partial displacement; 4, complete fracture with full displacement.

## Femur (shaft)

The femur is the largest and longest bone in the skeleton. The femoral head articulates with the acetabulum, and distally the femur ends with two large articular condyles that form the knee joint with tibial plateaux. Anteriorly it articulates with the patella. The medial condyle is more prominent than the lateral condyle.

Routine radiographic examination of the femur consists of anteroposterior and lateral views. When assessing the femur it is important to include the whole bone on the radiograph in order to assess for any rotation of the distal fragment. The knee joint must always be included. Major vascular injury is more common in distal femur fractures than in fractures occurring in the shaft, but nevertheless comminuted shaft fractures can result in a loss of 1–2 litres of blood into the soft tissues during the first 4 hours, producing clinical shock in some patients.

## Knee injuries

The knee joint consists of the femoral and tibial condyles, patella, internal and external ligaments including cruciate and collateral ligaments, menisci, and several bursae. A fabella is commonly seen lying in the lateral head of the gastrocnemius muscle which is posterolateral to the knee, and this sesamoid bone should not be mistaken for a fracture fragment.

The knee is commonly injured in motor vehicle accidents as well as in sporting activities. The routine radiographic views include anteroposterior and lateral views, and on occasion supplementary oblique views are required to identify tibial plateau fractures. If patellar injuries are suspected, then a skyline view is also obtained, which allows the patella to be viewed tangentially. In the anteroposterior projection of the knee, the patella is obscured by distal femur.

Tibial spine fractures are not common but when present may be associated with cruciate ligament injury, and a tunnel (intercondylar) view may be required to demonstrate these fractures adequately. In addition, the tunnel view is useful for assessing osteochondral fractures and intra-articular loose bodies as there is much less superimposition with the condyles.

As in other parts of the extremities, extensive soft-tissue damage including vascular injury may occur without any recognizable radiographic sign, and careful clinical inspection should always precede radiographic examination, even in patients with splintage applied.

CT with three-dimensional reformation is used in confirming suspected fractures, or to better define the extent and spatial relationships of fracture fragments around the knee. Although MRI is excellent in identifying soft-tissue injuries including ligamentous structures, it is currently not widely used as part of the emergency imaging of extremities.

Supracondylar, intercondylar, and condylar fractures of the femur are often due to direct trauma from a fall or blow to the distal femur.

The routine radiographs alone would be sufficient to identify these fractures in most cases.

Tibial plateau fractures are commonly produced by direct force on the tibia by the femoral condyles, and the lateral plateau is more often the side that is fractured. The fracture, when associated with depression of 5 mm or more, will inevitably require surgical management. Occasionally, CT may be necessary when routine films fail to demonstrate the degree of depression or displacement of the fracture fragments.

Sometimes a fracture line may be difficult to elicit and can only be suspected from a cross-table lateral radiograph that demonstrates a fat–fluid level of lipohaemarthrosis in the suprapatellar pouch. This usually indicates intra-articular extension of the fracture.

Apparently minor abnormalities on plain radiographs may be deceptive. For example, a Segond fracture is seen on the radiograph as a small vertical avulsion injury of the lateral aspect of the proximal lateral tibia. However, it is nearly always associated with injuries to the lateral collateral ligament and tears of the anterior cruciate ligament.

Dislocation of the knee joint is rare but represents a true orthopaedic emergency. Gross ligamentous disruption is involved and very often reduction occurs spontaneously, which makes early detection of its severe complications difficult. These include a high incidence of popliteal artery and peroneal nerve injuries. Therefore, clinical assessment becomes essential and radiographic examination is only complementary in these cases.

## Patella

The patella is a triangular sesamoid bone, which like all sesamoid bones develops in a tendon. In the case of the patella this is the quadriceps femoris tendon. Radiographic examination of the patella includes the anteroposterior, lateral, and special tangential (skyline) views.

Fractures to the patella commonly occur either from a direct blow or forceful contraction of the quadriceps muscles. Occasionally, difficulty can be encountered in differentiating fractures of the patella from two normal variants (bipartite or multipartite patella) on a single plain radiograph. The bipartite patella segments are normally located in the upper lateral quadrant of the patella and frequently occur in both knees. Fortunately fractures of the patella are associated with soft-tissue changes, such as fluid in the suprapatellar pouch, and are usually clinically evident. Therefore, differentiating them from bipartite patella is not always difficult when clinical and radiographic features are considered together. In the presence of a recent or suspected fracture of the patella, the knee should not be flexed.

## Tibia and fibula (shaft)

The upper end of the tibia articulates with the femoral condyles. While the lower medial end of the tibia forms the medial malleolus, the lateral aspect articulates with the fibula, and the inferior margin of the bone forms part of the ankle mortise. The shaft of the tibia has a superficial border that is covered only by the skin, and in cases of direct injury with significant force, open fractures commonly occur.

The proximal aspect of the fibula articulates with the lateral condyle of the tibia. Distally, it terminates as the lateral malleolus, which forms part of the ankle mortise. The tibia and fibula are held together just above the ankle mortise by the inferior tibiofibular ligaments, and when these are ruptured, parting or diastasis of the two bones may occur, which is radiologically evident as a widening of the mortise.

The type of fracture depends on the mechanism of injury. Direct trauma typically results in transverse and often comminuted fractures to either or both of the tibial and fibular shafts. Falls associated with a rotational force usually lead to oblique or spiral fractures. Torsion may be applied to the tibia in many sports, including football, skating, and skiing.

Fractures of the tibia and fibula usually occur in combination with ligament injuries or fractures about the knee or ankle. Radiological evaluation should therefore include the entire length of the tibia and fibula, including the knee and ankle on the same film, to detect either a fracture remote from the injury site or a rotational deformity.

Routine radiographs include the anteroposterior and lateral views. Oblique views may be necessary to identify subtle fractures, particularly in children when a single view may not show any abnormality and the other view shows only equivocal evidence of an undisplaced fracture.

## Ankle

The ankle is a complex joint formed by the distal end of the tibia and fibula and the upper articulating surface of the talus, as well as numerous surrounding ligamentous structures. The ankle mortise is formed by the medial and lateral malleoli together with the distal articulating surface of the tibia. The ankle mortise articulates with talus. The normal ankle joint space shows parallelism of the articular margins. Accessory bones of the ankle region may be seen, the most common being the os trigonum, found over the medial surface of the talus.

Ligaments around the ankle joint ensure stability. Often the presence of a specific ligamentous injury about the ankle can be inferred from the location and orientation of malleolar fractures. The lateral group of ligaments consists of the anterior and posterior talofibular ligaments, together with the calcaneofibular ligament, and the medial collateral (deltoid) ligament forms the medial component.

The routine radiographic views for the ankle include the antero-posterior (straight) and lateral views. However, in the straight antero-posterior view, the distal fibula (lateral malleolus) overlaps the lateral aspect of the body of the talus, making the talofibular joint space difficult to see adequately.

In the lateral view, the malleoli are projected over one another. This view clearly demonstrates the talotibial joint, anterior and posterior lips of the medial malleolus, and the lateral malleolus. An oblique view of the ankle is usually obtained when the lateral malleolus and tibiofibular joint require more careful evaluation.

When the patient's condition permits, a mortise view can be obtained by internally rotating the foot 15–20°, thereby placing the malleoli in the same horizontal plane. Identification of any mortise abnormality is one of the most important aspects in the evaluation of an ankle fracture or dislocation. Asymmetry may be the only evidence of significant ligamentous injury.

With severe ligamentous injury, a dislocation of the ankle in a lateral or medial direction may occur. This typically occurs in combination with fractures of both malleoli.

Often the kind of fracture to the malleoli will reflect the direction of the forces causing injury. For instance, a horizontal fracture generally occurs on the side to which the force is applied and an oblique fracture occurs on the opposite side. Inversion injuries tend to produce a transverse lateral malleolus fracture and an oblique medial malleolus fracture. Eversion injuries produce the directly opposite pattern.

It is essential to look for evidence of associated proximal fractures with ankle injuries. High fibular fracture may occur in external rotational ankle injuries with rupture of the anterior talofibular ligament and a tear of the interosseous membrane. This injury may be easily missed as the presentation will be masked by the prominent clinical findings around the ankle. This combination of injury has been termed as Maisonneuve fracture. It is essential to include examination of the upper fibula in all clinical examinations of the injured ankle.

A set of rules has been evaluated in Canada and Hong Kong to assist clinicians in deciding the need for ankle radiographs. These are known as the Ottawa ankle rules. An ankle X-ray series is only necessary if there is pain near the malleoli and any of these findings:

(1)  inability to bear weight both immediately and in A&E department (four steps); or

(2)  bone tenderness at the posterior edge or tip of either malleolus.

A foot X-ray series is only necessary if there is pain in the midfoot and any of these findings:

(1) inability to bear weight both immediately and in A&E department (four steps); or

(2) bone tenderness at the navicular or the base of the fifth metatarsal.

## Foot and heel

The foot (Fig. 16.12) is anatomically divided into the hindfoot (heel), consisting of the calcaneus and talus; midfoot, containing the navicular, cuboid, and three cuneiforms; and the forefoot, made up of the metatarsals and phalanges. Variable sesamoid bones are also present, the most frequently identified of which is the peroneal sesamoid, found between the cuboid and the base of the fifth metatarsal.

The routine radiographic views are separated into two regions in which additional specific radiographic views may also be required. For the foot, the routine radiographic projections include the anteroposterior and the internally rotated oblique views (Fig. 16.13). The internally rotated oblique view projects the third (lateral) cuneiform, cuboid, and lateral three metatarsal bones in profile, which would otherwise be superimposed. To visualize the entire tarsus, the anteroposterior view of both the foot and ankle are required. The lateral view is of limited use as bones of the midfoot and forefoot are superimposed on each other, although the subtalar joint, talonavicular, and calcaneocuboid joints are well seen on this view.

For the heel, the routine radiographic views are the lateral and axial views. Bohler's angle is determined on the lateral view, and is measured at the intersection of lines drawn tangentially to the anterior and posterior aspects of the superior surface of the calcaneus. This angle normally ranges between 28° and 40°. An angle less than 28° is abnormal and suggests a depressed fracture of the subtalar portion of the calcaneus. The axial view of the calcaneus demonstrates the posterior two-thirds of the calcaneus well and can confirm cortical breaks not easily detected on the lateral view.

### Hindfoot: talus and calcaneum

#### Talus
The talus articulates with the ankle mortise, the calcaneus inferiorly, and the navicular anteriorly. Its articulation with the tibia is weight bearing.

CT with three-dimensional reformatting capability is useful in

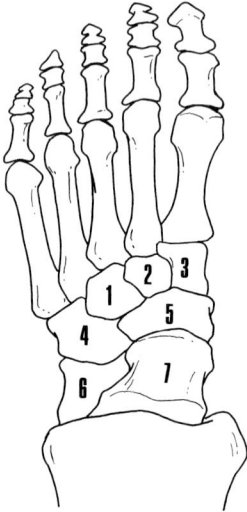

**Fig. 16.12** Foot, dorsi-plantar view: 1, 2, 3, cuneiforms; 4, cuboid; 5, navicular; 6, calcaneum; 7, talus.

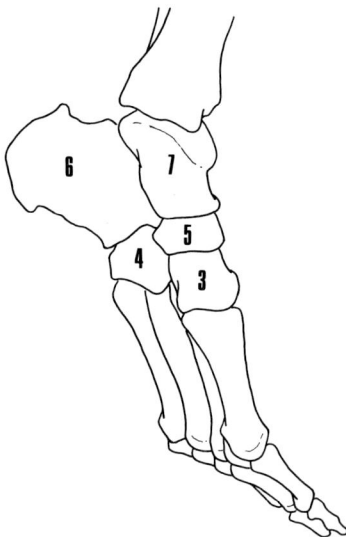

**Fig. 16.13** Foot, oblique view: 3, cuneiform; 4, cuboid; 5, navicular; 6, calcaneum; 7, talus.

demonstrating subtle talar neck fractures and the alignment of fragments. MRI is better in defining osteochondral fracture of the talar dome, and may be useful when available.

### Calcaneus

The calcaneus forms the heel of the foot and is the largest of the tarsal bones. It articulates with the talus superiorly and anteromedially, and with the cuboid anteriorly.

Calcaneal fractures (Fig. 16.14) are the most common foot fractures encountered. They usually result from a fall from height and the mechanism of injury is usually compression. These injuries may be associated with fractures of the thoracolumbar spine as well as vertical shear injuries of the pelvis. On occasion, clinical evidence of calcaneal fracture may be present but difficult to demonstrate on the plain radiographs despite careful assessment of the cortical margins and trabecular detail. In such cases CT may be necessary to demonstrate the fracture and the degree of articular surface involvement.

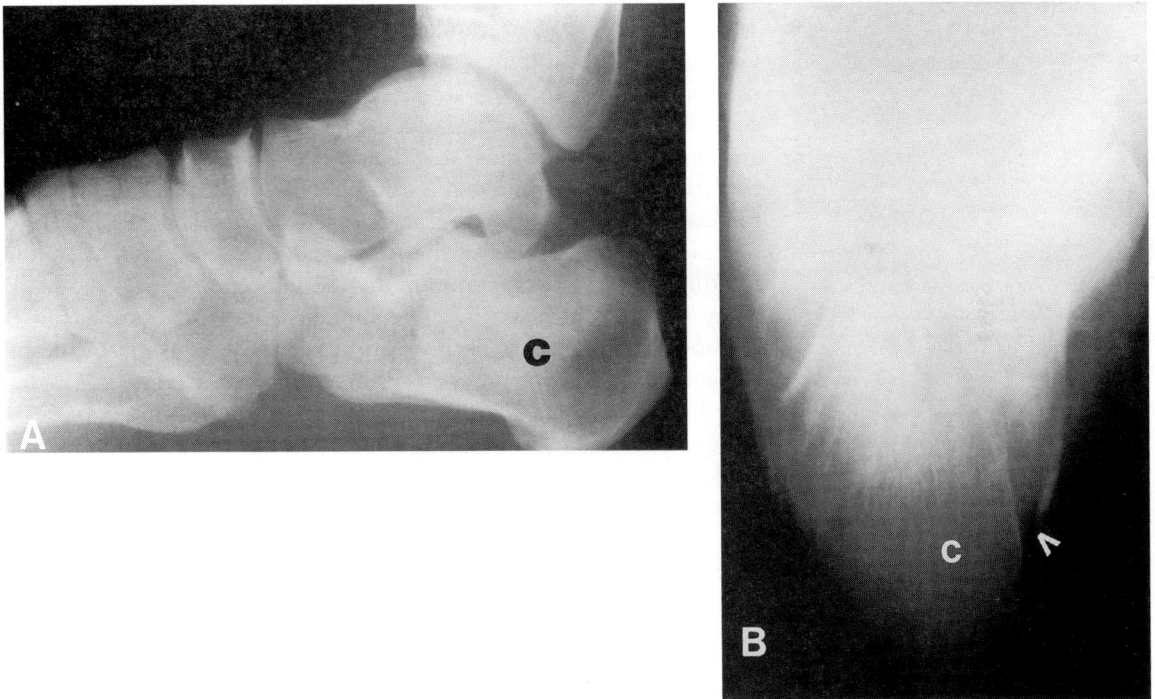

**Fig. 16.14** Calcaneum, fracture. (A) Lateral view; calcaneal fracture with loss of normal Bohler's angle. (B) Axial view; <, discontinuity of calcaneal cortices.

## Midfoot: navicular, cuboid, and cuneiform

Isolated midfoot fractures are uncommon but this region is most susceptible to direct trauma because it is the least mobile part of the foot. Often, injuries are difficult to detect radiographically but, taken together with clinical information concerning the most tender site, most routine radiographic views taken of foot can help establish a diagnosis.

## Forefoot: metatarsals and phalanges

In the foot, there are five metatarsal bones that articulate with the phalanges anteriorly and the tarsus posteriorly. The first metatarsal is the shortest and thickest while the second is the longest. Each toe has three phalanges, with the exception of the big toe that has two instead. Sesamoid bones of the foot are numerous and varied.

Fractures of the small bones of the foot are uncommon in multiple trauma victims, but when present are often overlooked in the face of more obvious and life-threatening conditions elsewhere. Injuries to these areas, however, also need to be identified early, as they may lead to chronic morbidity and delay the ultimate recovery of the patient.

Lisfranc fracture dislocation of the tarsometatarsal junction (Fig. 16.15) may often be overlooked. The injury occurs in extreme abrupt abduction of the forefoot as the result of severe direct or indirect trauma. On the anteroposterior view the normal alignment of the second metatarsal and the middle cuneiform is almost invariable lost and thus suggests the diagnosis. There are variations, but careful attention paid to the alignment and orientation of the tarsal and metatarsal bones will ensure that these fractures are identified successfully.

Fractures of the base of the fifth metatarsal (also known as Jones fractures) are the most common metatarsal injuries (Fig. 16.16A, B). They may be produced by either direct or indirect trauma, but the common mechanism is an inversion injury with avulsion of the fifth metatarsal base by the peroneus brevis tendon attached to it. The fracture line is orientated in a transverse manner, contrasting with the obliquely orientated apophyseal line seen during childhood and adolescence (Fig. 16.16C).

Injuries to the metatarsals and phalanges are not difficult to identify. In most cases, the routine radiographic views, including the anteroposterior and oblique views, are sufficient to detect fractures.

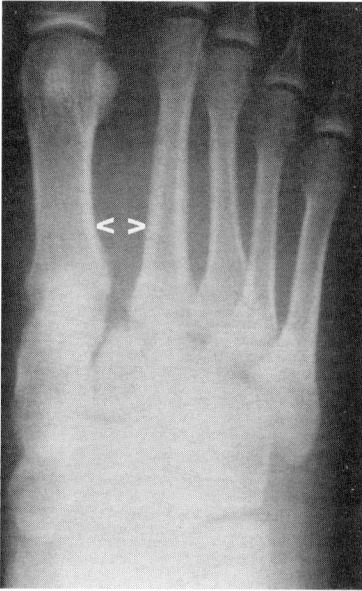

**Fig. 16.15** Foot, dorsiplantar view, Lisfranc fracture dislocation: < >, wide separation of the first and second metatarsals.

# PAEDIATRIC INJURIES

Skeletal trauma in children warrants special attention because in many situations the type, pattern, and distribution of fractures is quite

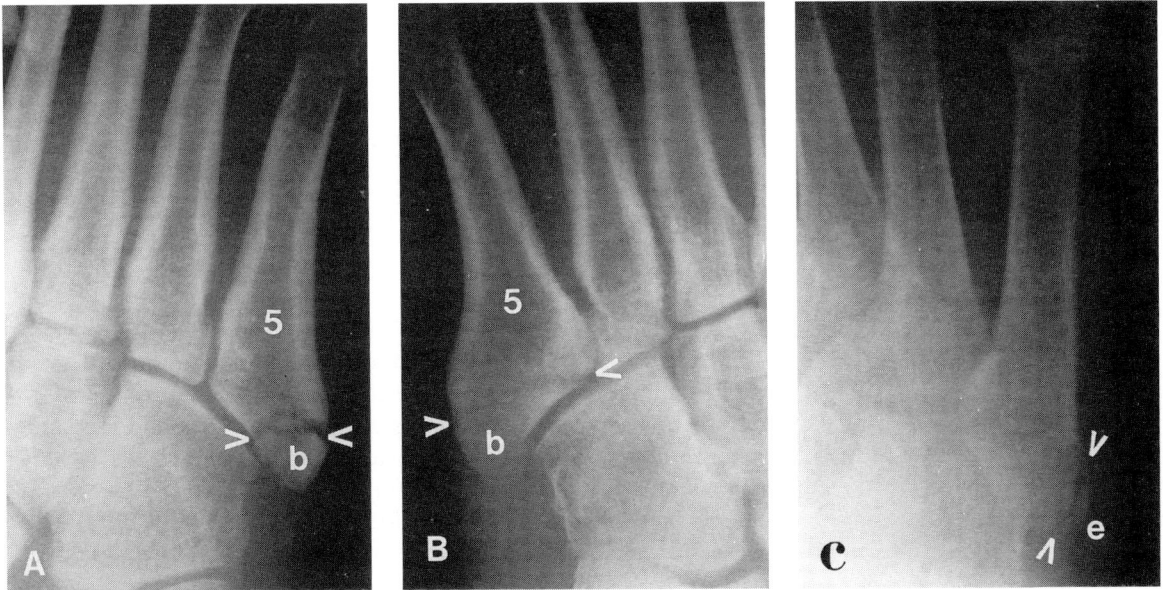

**Fig. 16.16** Foot, dorsiplantar view. (A and B) Jones fracture; ><, horizontally orientated fracture line across the base of the fifth metatarsal (5); b, fracture fragment. (C) Unfused apophysis; v, apophyseal lucent line is almost vertically orientated and almost parallels the long axis of the fifth metatarsal.

different from those commonly encountered in the adults, even if the mechanism of injury appears the same. Also, developmental changes may be confusing and lead to errors in diagnosis.

The pattern of fractures differs from that in adults due to the presence of growth plates. When a child reaches the age of 15 or 16 years, the epiphyseal plates are about to close or have already closed and bony injuries then resemble those of the adult population. Dislocations are uncommon in children but, if they do occur, these commonly involve the elbow. Ligamentous injuries in children are extremely infrequent.

As always, an adequate clinical history, including the mechanism of injury coupled with the clinical findings of the site of maximal tenderness and presence of swelling, ensures that subtle fractures are not missed.

Very occasionally, comparison views may be taken when there is a difficulty in ascertaining if the questioned abnormality is a normal variant. This practice is to be discouraged as a routine, since there are atlases available for quick reference. Frequent radiographs taken for comparison would expose children to unnecessary additional radiation.

Other imaging modalities may be used to demonstrate injuries that are difficult to detect on plain radiographs. These include isotope scans that are sensitive and can identify fractures as early as 1 day after the injury, but unfortunately are not specific. Complex joint fractures are best evaluated by CT, which has an added advantage of being able to perform two- or three-dimensional reformatted images. MRI, because of the limitations mentioned earlier, has yet to find a clear role.

## Type of fractures

Incomplete fractures, including buckle, greenstick, and bowing fractures, are common in children. Buckle or torus fractures result from abnormal sharp angulation, and show an irregularity and incomplete break in one side of the bone cortex. The opposite cortex is usually intact. The greenstick fracture, on the other hand, has a break in one side of the cortex but the other side is intact. Acute bowing fractures are seen as an abnormal curvature of a long bone, often with no visible break in the cortex.

Growth plates are common sites of injury. Under the common and widely used Salter–Harris classification, growth-plate injuries are divided into five types. In type I, the fracture line passes through the growth or epiphyseal plate. In type II, the fracture line extends through the growth plate and into the metaphysis (this is the most frequent type). In type III, the fracture line extends through the growth plate and into the epiphysis. In type IV, the fracture line extends through the metaphysis, across and occasionally along the growth plate, and then through the epiphysis. Type V injuries, instead of showing a fracture line, demonstrate crushing of all or part of the growth plate. This type of fracture is rare and may be associated with subsequent arrested bone growth.

## Complications

Complications are uncommon because most paediatric fractures heal well. However, the most important complication, with possible long-term morbidity, involves fracture of the growth plate. Failure to identify these fractures early may lead to delays in treatment, resulting in growth disturbance. Despite treatment, fracture of the growth plate may cause premature fusion, leading to limb length discrepancy. When just one of the two epiphyses at the end of a long bone is fractured (e.g. the lower humerus), growth arrest of that epiphysis may lead to angular deformity in the limb as the normal one continues to grow.

# Upper limb

## The shoulder

The most common bony injury around the shoulder is a fracture of the clavicle, usually due to a fall on the outstretched arm or a direct fall on the shoulder. The middle third of the clavicle is the common site of injury and this generally heals well without any noticeable morbidity. Return to normal activity is quite rapid.

Acromioclavicular joint separation is rare during childhood, but epiphyseal injuries around the ends may occur.

Scapular fractures and shoulder dislocations are uncommon but may occur in severe trauma, as in motor vehicle accidents.

## Humerus

The second most common injury around the shoulder in children is a fracture of the surgical neck of the humerus. The normal appearance of the proximal humeral growth plate may seem wide and may be mistaken for a fracture.

## Elbow

In general, dislocations of joints are uncommon in children, except in the elbow region. The mechanism is usually a hyperextension injury, resulting in posterior dislocation with either some medial or lateral displacement. These injuries may be accompanied by positive anterior and posterior fat pad signs which are identified on a lateral view of the elbow. This indicates the presence of a joint effusion or haemarthrosis.

Avulsion of the medial epicondyle is frequently associated with elbow dislocation. Displacement of more than 2 mm would be considered significant and usually requires orthopaedic management.

In children and adolescents, it is important to consider the normal chronological sequence of the appearance of the ossification of the distal growth centres (Table 16.1) so as to recognize injuries to these structures. In evaluating the elbow, the abnormal presence or absence of bony structures not conforming to the child's chronological age sequence may suggest a displaced fracture fragment. An example would be when the lateral epicondyle but not the medial epicondyle is found on the radiograph. This suggests that an avulsion fracture of the medial epicondyle has occurred, commonly resulting from a valgus injury of the elbow. Effort should be made to locate the displaced fracture fragment, which may be some distance away from its normal position.

**Table 16.1** Age of appearance of ossification centres

| Ossification centres | Age of appearance (years) |
| --- | --- |
| Capitellum | 2 |
| Medial epicondyle | 4 |
| Trochlea | 8 |
| Lateral epicondyle | 10 |

## Supracondylar fractures

The most common mechanism of injury is a fall on the outstretched arm. When the distal fragment is displaced, it invariably displaces dorsally. The displaced supracondylar fracture in a child is an emergency because of the risk of associated vascular compromise of the forearm muscles and hand. The radial pulse must be checked immediately and observed regularly.

There may be only minimal displacement of the distal fragment of the fracture, thus making the diagnosis difficult. Fortunately there are radiological clues: the presence of a joint effusion, evident from a positive anterior and posterior fat pad, as described earlier, is an important start. Next, the anterior humeral line is drawn down from the anterior aspect of the shaft of the humerus on a true lateral radiograph. This should pass through the middle of the ossification centre of the lateral condyle or capitellum in the normal elbow. However, if the anterior humeral line instead passes through anteriorly or, less infrequently, posteriorly this usually would imply the presence of a supracondylar fracture.

## Lateral condyle

Injuries to the lateral condyle are the second most common injury to occur around the paediatric elbow after supracondylar fractures. Fractures almost invariably pass through the unossified portion of the distal humeral epiphysis.

## Ulna and radius

Fractures of the radial neck can occur throughout childhood, but fractures of the proximal ulna are uncommon. Both usually occur as a result of a fall on the outstretched arm.

Diaphyseal (midshaft) fractures are frequently of the incomplete type in young children. This is the most common site for acute bowing fractures, but in older children fractures are more often complete. An isolated ulnar shaft fracture with external bruising may indicate a defensive injury, and child abuse must be considered.

Monteggia fractures often occur from mild trauma while Galeazzi fractures rarely occur in children. Monteggia fracture describes a combination of ulnar fracture with dislocation of the proximal radio-ulnar joint. Galeazzi fractures occur when fracture of the radius is associated with dislocation of the distal radio-ulnar joint.

Fractures occurring at the distal end of the radius and ulna are common. Again, the mechanism of injury is the result of a fall on the outstretched hand. The distal fragment is usually dorsally displaced. Occasionally, epiphyseal fractures may not be obvious but may be evident from an indirect sign. This is the positive pronator quadratus fat pad sign, which is due to haematoma from the fracture displacing the fat pad anteriorly over the palmar aspect of the distal forearm. Normally this fat pad is not separated from the distal radius by more than 7 mm in females and 10 mm in males. A good lateral view of the region is essential in order to detect abnormalities of the pad.

### Hand and carpus

Injuries in these regions are uncommon, except perhaps dislocation of the fingers in older children and fingertip injuries involving the terminal phalanges in smaller children.

## Lower limb

### Femur

Most fractures of the femur occur in the middle third. In the younger child the fracture is usually of the greenstick type. If this occurs during infancy without a credible history from the accompanying parent or guardian, the injury should raise the possibility of child abuse. In older children these fractures are frequently associated with more serious trauma, including motor vehicle accidents. In most instances injuries from these high-energy transfers present as complete fractures.

Some late complications include leg length discrepancy, which may lead to functional morbidity.

Fractures of the proximal and distal ends of the femur are uncommon in children. Proximal femur fractures usually involve the neck more frequently than the subtrochanteric region, while intertrochanteric fractures are rare. The most common fracture of the distal femoral epiphysis is usually a type II epiphyseal fracture.

### Knee

Fractures about the knee are encountered more often than significant ligamentous injuries, with meniscal injuries occurring less frequently than in the adult population. Although patellar fractures are uncommon, they and avulsion of the anterior tibial spine together represent most of the fractures seen around the knee in children. In the case of avulsion of the anterior tibial spine, the lateral view of the knee shows the fracture best.

Traumatic dislocation of the patella occurs infrequently, and it should be remembered that, as in adults, the patella often reduces to its normal position by the time the patient is seen by the examining physician in the A&E department.

Proximal tibial growth-plate injuries are uncommon and occur less frequently than injuries to the distal femoral growth plate. Most of these fractures are found in adolescents.

In children who complain of knee pain which seems disproportionate to the clinical and radiographic examination findings in the knee, the hip should be examined, since pain from abnormality of the hip may be referred distally.

### Leg

The most common lower extremity injuries in children are those of the tibial and fibular shafts, usually resulting from a twisting mechanism, but also occasionally from direct trauma. Isolated fibular fractures are uncommon. Generally, fractures of either bone heal well when no angular deformity exists. Stress fractures of the tibia are seen commonly in the upper third. 'Toddler fractures' usually occur as spiral fractures of the tibial shaft, and often present with non-specific symptoms, including reluctance of the child to walk.

### Ankle

In children ligamentous injuries are uncommon compared to fractures around the epiphyseal plates, generally due to the fact that the ligaments are stronger than bones in this region.

The most common fractures around the ankle in a child are type I fractures of the distal fibula and type II fractures of the distal tibia. When the fractures are undisplaced, the presence of an ankle joint effusion may be the only radiological clue. This is seen as a round or triangular soft-tissue density displacing the fat pad anteriorly at the level of the ankle joint.

When more complex injuries occur, CT is generally required for further evaluation.

### Foot

In the foot, metatarsal fractures are common in children. These often occur at the base of the fifth metatarsal, but should not be confused with the normal appearances of the epiphysis at this location.

# BIBLIOGRAPHY

Ballinger PW. Merrill's Atlas of Radiographic Positions and Radiologic Procedures, 8th edn. Missouri: Mosby, 1995; 1:37–270.

Bledsore RE, Izenmark JL. Displacement of fat pads in disease and injury at the elbow. Radiology 1959; 73:717.

Brawner BD, Jupiter JB, Levine Am, Trafton PG. Skeletal Trauma: Fractures, Dislocations, Ligamentous injuries. Philadelphia: WB Saunders, 1992.

Callander CL. Surgical Anatomy, 2nd edn. Philadelphia: WB Saunders, 1950.

De Palma AF. The Management of Fractures and Dislocations, 2nd edn. Philadelphia: WB Saunders, 1970.

Gilula LA. The Traumatised Hand and Wrist: Radiographic and Anatomic Correlation. Philadelphia: WB Saunders, 1992.

Grainger RG, Allison DJ. Diagnostic Radiology, 2nd edn. Edinburgh: Churchill Livingstone, 1992.

Helms CA. Fundamentals of Skeletal Radiology. Philadelphia: WB Saunders, 1989.

Kaye J. Fractures and dislocations of the hand and wrist. Semin Roentgenol 1978; 13:109.

Keats TE, Pope TL. The acromioclavicular joint: normal variation and the diagnosis of dislocation. Skeletal Radiol 1988; 17:159–62.

Leffers D. Dislocations and soft tissue injuries of the knee. In: Browner BD, Jupiter JB, Levine AM, Trafton PG, eds. Skeletal Trauma; Fractures, Dislocations, Ligamentous Injuries. Philadelphia: WB Saunders, 1992; 1724–5.

McCort JJ. Trauma Radiology. New York: Churchill Livingstone, 1990.

McGahan JP, Rob GT, Dublin A. Fractures of the scapula. J Trauma 1980; 20:880–3.

Meschan IA. An Atlas of Anatomy Basic to Radiology. Philadelphia: WB Saunders, 1975.

Park WM, Hughes SPF, eds. Orthopaedic Radiology. Oxford: Blackwell Scientific Publications, 1987.

Pavlov H, Freiberger RH. Fractures and dislocations about the shoulder. Semin Roentgenol 1978; 13:85.

Ralston EL. Handbook of Fractures. St Louis: CV Mosby, 1967.

Rogers LF. Elbow. In: Roentgenology of Fractures and Dislocations. New York: Grune & Stratton, 1978.

Salter RB. Textbook of Disorders and Injuries of the Musculoskeletal System. Baltimore: Williams & Wilkins, 1970.

# PART 4
## *Training, audit, and the future*

# CHAPTER 17

# Education, training, and audit

The theme of this book has been to emphasize the rational use of imaging in the light of good clinical assessment. A good introductory course for Senior House Officers in Accident and Emergency, and their subsequent in-service training, should include the skills of clinical examination and film assessment in an integrated way.

The outcome and efficiency of education and training must also be measured. This measurement is more meaningful if it relates to real clinical practice rather than a classroom examination, and although it is relatively easy to set a test in which doctors are expected to identify abnormalities on radiographs, good results in such tests provide little reassurance that the doctor is effective in clinical practice. One of the best ways of monitoring practice on an ongoing basis is by clinical audit. Methods of organizing this will be discussed later in this chapter.

## EDUCATION

Education in the use of imaging in trauma is an integral part of general education in the clinical management of A&E patients, not a separate discipline. Imaging has a defined place within the teaching of patient management, but should not be considered separate from it.

## TRAINING

Bearing in mind what has been said above concerning the need for integration, the training of accident and emergency doctors does require coverage of some specific skills. Teaching these skills requires access to certain equipment and resources.

### A teaching room

Every A&E department should have a quiet room that can be blacked out for the purpose of showing teaching slides, and which is also equipped with an X-ray viewing box (preferably several). The room should also be provided with a full-sized skeleton mounted on a stand and perhaps some disarticulated bones and models of key organs as well.

Preferably, the teaching room should be located within the A&E department itself, so that staff on duty can be included in the tutorial if operational considerations permit.

## A departmental film library

It is relatively easy in any busy A&E department to accumulate a stock of teaching films covering the common disorders, specifically for trauma and also for emergency medicine in general. The problem with such collections is that they need to be labelled and indexed to a high standard in order to be useful.

This collection is of sufficient importance that most radiology departments will consider making copies of the original patient films, provided that this is seen as a joint venture. If cost considerations are paramount, 35 mm slides are an economical alternative to duplicating the X-ray films. While it is best for optimum results to send the films to a medical illustration department for slide-making, adequate results can be achieved using a standard viewing box and a 35 mm camera with a black-and-white slide film. Colour-slide film also produces acceptable results, but the images tend to develop a blue hue with age. If slides are made in the A&E department using a standard viewing box, the bright areas of screen surrounding the X-ray film should be covered with masking paper to avoid problems with inaccurate exposure.

Each X-ray film or slide should be given a label and index number which can be cross-referenced to a card index or similar filing system containing clinical details, diagnosis, and teaching highlights. If a filing cabinet can be devoted to the index, clinical photographs and data can be added to the materials in order to build up complete problem-orientated case presentations.

In addition to the films covering abnormalities, it is advantageous to have a complete set of normal radiographs of the whole skeleton, including common normal variations. Since most radiographs taken for trauma turn out to be normal, building up this part of the library should prove to be the most straightforward. Age variations will need to be included, including the epiphyses at different ages for key areas, such as the hand, foot, and all of the major joints.

Increasingly over the next decade, A&E departments will acquire digital radiology systems, and doctors will routinely view their radiographs on a computer monitor rather than as a film on an X-ray box. The A&E department needs to be involved at an early stage with the planning of PACS (picture archiving and communication systems) and digital radiology systems in order to derive the maximum benefit from them. It is possible with forward planning to set up an image library as a separate resource on a digital radiology system, which can store not only radiographs, but also reports and educational information in text form. These facilities should be discussed with the manufacturer as part of the system specification, at the time of planning, rather than as something to be added later after the system is commissioned.

The compilation of an image library requires persistence and enthusiasm, and it is best to make the task a responsibility of a small number of keen operational staff. Perhaps one of the best ways of making a start is to encourage all staff to keep a simple record of the name, image type, and findings of specific cases in a 'library book' placed within the clinical area of the A&E department. This avoids interesting radiographs being detained in unspecified locations or being lost from the system. Once every month or two, the 'library staff' can ask the clerical staff to obtain the X-ray films from file, and a meeting can be held to decide which films need to be copied. The patients' clinical details can also be drawn from file at the same time, and a folder to receive the materials is set up within the library. Once all the details are collated, it is best for the name of the patient to be deleted from the teaching materials for confidentiality.

# AUDIT

Safety net details were discussed in Part 1 of this book, and these systems can form the basis of the audit of imaging in trauma.

In all cases where the radiologist's report differs from the patient diagnosis, audit should take place. There might be several reasons for such a discrepancy. First, the accident and emergency doctor may have genuinely failed to spot a radiological abnormality, or may have diagnosed an abnormality where none really exists. Secondly, the abnormality may have been seen but appropriate management not given. Thirdly, the abnormality may not relate to the present injury, and the clinician has failed to convey to the radiologist a history of previous injury or an accurate description of the precise body site involved. Lastly, and fortunately rarely, the radiologist may not be correct in diagnosing the abnormality.

A further category of cases, which initially escape the safety net, includes those in which the radiological abnormality is missed by both the A&E doctor and by the radiologist. Such patients may present later with ongoing problems or complications arising from the injury. If cases of this nature are identified, they should also be subject to audit.

The process of audit is assisted by applying a scoring system to the missed or misdiagnosed injuries. Such injuries can be grouped into the following categories:

1.  The abnormalities are not apparently clinically significant, and do not require a change in patient management. No further contact with the patient is required.

2.  The abnormalities are not apparently clinically significant, and do not require a change in patient management, but further contact with the patient and explanation of the abnormality is required for reassurance.

3.  The abnormality is clinically significant, suggesting the need for a change of management or mode of follow-up. Further clinical contact with the patient is required urgently, preferably on the same day.

4.  The abnormality is clinically significant, suggesting the need for a change of management or mode of follow-up. Further clinical contact with the patient is required, but follow-up is not so urgent and can be organized as an elective follow-up clinic attendance (e.g. A&E review clinic).

5.  The abnormality appears to be unrelated to the current injury, but requires follow-up.

6.  The abnormality does not appear to be related to the current injury, and does not require follow-up.

7.  There is uncertainty whether the radiological abnormality truly exists, and further discussion is required before deciding on follow-up.

8.  The images have been reported as normal by the radiologist but as abnormal by the A&E doctor. The treatment given has been inappropriate, and the patient requires follow-up for re-examination (e.g. the patient may have a missed soft-tissue injury rather than a bony one).

9.  The images have been reported as normal by the radiologist but an abnormality has been diagnosed by the accident and emergency doctor. However, treatment is appropriate for the injury, and no reason exists for early recall of the patient or for a change of management at this time.

10.  The images taken are inappropriate for the adequate diagnosis of the problem, and the patient needs to be recalled for further investigation.

A classification system such as this provides a framework for both the further clinical management of the patient, and for education and review. As mentioned in Chapter 3, many medico-legal problems may be avoided if diagnostic errors are corrected rapidly and with minimal discomfort and inconvenience to the patient. In addition, such errors can be viewed as a learning experience and treated in a positive light, the experience being shared with all staff in a non-threatening way. Since it is entirely predictable that some errors by inexperienced medical staff will occur, the audit provides a good test of the adequacy of management procedures for minimizing the harmful effects of such incidents.

All instances of missed imaging diagnosis should be fed back to the individual doctor who has treated the patient, but in addition some salient cases can be discussed weekly or monthly in the departmental meeting (preferably with the doctor and patient remaining anonymous) in order that all of the staff can benefit from the lessons learned. All minutes of audit meetings should be kept confidential and should not contain identifying details.

# CHAPTER 18

# *New techniques and the future*

## PRESENT AND FUTURE

Since the discovery of X-rays in 1895, advances in imaging technology for medical diagnostic purposes have been astounding. These advances have found their way towards new clinical applications that have helped to revolutionize the practice of accident and emergency medicine and trauma care.

## CONVENTIONAL RADIOGRAPHY

Plain radiographic imaging has undergone vast improvement over the years and now gives clearer images with lower doses of radiation. Conventional radiography remains the 'backbone' of patient evaluation, but unfortunately, until recently, the quality of portable/bedside radiography has often been highly variable, despite the large number of portable examinations performed. This has been due largely to the less than ideal circumstances in which the film is obtained.

The advent of digital computed radiography (CR) has allowed some degree of post-acquisition image manipulation which may compensate for the shortcomings of portable radiography and can potentially improve the image quality, thus avoiding a repeat radiograph. CR has allowed some radiation-dose saving to patients, but also allows more consistency in the quality of both portable and general radiography.

A more recent development is the introduction of electronic and semiconductor technology to capture the latent image data directly to create a digital image, termed direct radiography (DR). CR uses a phosphor-based storage system, dependent on conversion of X-rays to light, whereas DR uses an amorphous selenium-coated thin-film transistor (TFT) array and converts X-ray energy directly to digital signals. The image can be previewed immediately on a workstation, printed as a hard copy display, stored, or be transmitted to other locations. However, as with any new technology, further clinical evaluation will be required to assess its full potential.

Both CR and DR technology are compatible with an all-digital environment, which will allow realization of the full benefit of the integration not only of radiological images and reports, but also of laboratory results and of the patient's previous data from hospital information systems.

# ULTRASONOGRAPHY

Three particular areas in which ultrasonography is being used increasingly are in the evaluation of haemoperitoneum, haemothorax, and haemopericardium. Because no ionizing radiation is involved, the use of this modality in pregnant patients is invaluable. Presently, most examinations performed in the A&E department are often 'target' orientated; for example, to assess for the presence or absence of haemoperitoneum in abdominal trauma and the need to transfer the patient to the operating theatre immediately. The sensitivity and specificity can be very high and ultrasound often avoids the need for diagnostic peritoneal lavage.

New advances in sonography have increased its application in the A&E department, and may supplement, or in some cases replace, other difficult and often hazardous radiological examinations in a trauma victim. Pulse and colour Doppler, and the added sensitivity of directional colour angiography (DCA), are presently available and are being improved for the evaluation of vascular injuries.

Currently, emergency physicians learning to use ultrasonography have to recognize organs examined in two-dimensional images, and this often requires a significant amount of training. However, some currently available imaging techniques such as Siescape from Siemens have an image-processor algorithm that processes data in real time and blends successive ultrasound images together to display them in a single, large, composite image. This allows large organs and vessels to be viewed in their entire extent.

The promise of real-time three-dimensional images in the near future with the aid of supercomputer processors, allowing rapid processing of ultrasound signals, will undoubtedly enable the operator to see more anatomy and pathology, and, more importantly, makes an ultrasonographic examination easier.

# COMPUTED TOMOGRAPHY

Whereas once the evaluation of soft-tissue injuries depended solely on clinical examination, the use of CT has revolutionized the investigation of visceral trauma, particularly of the brain. Its use has also reduced the number of negative exploratory operations, in particular laparotomies.

The availability of faster scanners has enabled critically ill patients to be imaged more quickly and ensures that urgent treatment can be given as soon as possible.

Helical (spiral) CT scan is faster and is becoming the method of choice, superseding conventional CT. The advantages of faster acquisition of volumetric data include allowing an entire body region to be scanned within a single breath-hold and reduction or elimination of respiratory misregistration, especially in uncooperative patients. Better multiplanar and three-dimensional reconstruction capabilities make it particularly useful in imaging musculoskeletal trauma.

The primary applications of helical CT are in patients with trauma of the chest, abdomen, and musculoskeletal system. Imaging of head injuries is often less demanding on the scanner and can be readily performed with a conventional CT.

As in other areas, advances in computer technology have brought virtual reality imaging into radiology, utilizing data from helical (spiral) CT. One such application is CT image reconstruction of the airway and its display as virtual reality endoscopy. Although still in their infancy in terms of development, virtual reality endoscopy images were found to be comparable to actual bronchoscopic findings in detecting pathology. Clinical applications of this technology may find their way to the A&E department in coming years.

Advances made with new techniques in three-dimensional CT angiography will eventually reduce our reliance on conventional angiography, which carries the added risks of invasive procedural complications. In addition, interventional procedures that were previously impractical can now be performed with the faster helical CT.

# MAGNETIC RESONANCE IMAGING

MRI is one of the more recently developed fields in radiology and has already been shown to provide excellent morphological images of the body organs. However, it has not really made an impact on the practice of A&E departments in terms of ready clinical applications. This is due largely to its limited availability, the long acquisition time required, lower accuracy for detecting fractures, and its limitations in terms of incompatibility with monitoring devices, image degradation due to patient's motion, and the question of high cost.

In head-injured patients, a CT scanner is able to detect the presence of intracranial haematomas which will require early surgical intervention, often in less than 5 minutes. Coupled with its wide availability, relative lack of contraindications, and high accuracy in detecting haemorrhage, this has made CT the diagnostic study of choice for the initial evaluation of head-injured patients in most centres. Although this is the case at present, MRI is now beginning to overcome some of its limitations.

It is currently possible to obtain high-quality $T_1$-weighted scans in 2–3 minutes using standard spin echo techniques to detect virtually all significant intracranial haematomas. Recently available echoplanar hardware and pulse sequences have made it possible to obtain $T_2$-weighted scans within seconds. Perhaps in the not too distant future, MRI may become a viable alternative for the initial evaluation of head-injured patients.

MRI of the thorax and abdomen has undergone much improvement since the beginning of its use. Technological developments include adaptation of the acquisition time to breath-holding, acquisition over multiple respiratory cycles, adjustment of the contrast of various sequences, and development of more sensitive receiver coils and faster gradient systems. It is expected that the overall sensitivity and specificity of MRI will further improve. The development of self-shielded magnets, wider and more accessible scanning gantries, and a wide range of non-ferromagnetic life-support and monitoring devices which are more compatible with the MRI environment, will greatly facilitate the evaluation of critically ill patients.

For vascular injuries, MRI angiography is emerging as a useful tool for the non-invasive evaluation of the cardiovascular system. Ultrafast echoplanar imaging (EPI) acquisition strategies are becoming more readily available, which often allow breath-hold acquisition of entire vascular territories and the exploitation of short-lived flow-enhancing measures. Potential EPI MRI angiography applications include carotid and renal arteries, the portal venous system, and arteries and veins of the limbs.

# INTERVENTIONAL RADIOLOGY

An increasing array of new interventional techniques has been developed to treat injuries sustained from major trauma, making use of percutaneous imaging-guided techniques, which are often used for both diagnosis and treatment.

Innovative techniques and further improvement in equipment, such as catheter design, stents, and embolic agents, have recently reduced the numbers of laparotomies and other surgical treatments.

Until recently, fluoroscopy and CT were the main imaging

modalities employed for interventional radiology. However, with advances made in MRI, and particularly MR angiography, the need for many conventional catheter angiograms has been reduced.

High-speed imaging methods that allow real-time imaging (fluoroscopic mode) is becoming routine and enables the use of MRI to guide interventional procedures. The use of multiplanar imaging has also enabled the establishment of virtual reality MRI operating suites.

# TELEMEDICINE, AND PICTURE ARCHIVING AND COMMUNICATION SYSTEMS (PACS)

Telemedicine and PACS are increasingly being implemented in many institutions. The American Telemedicine Association defines the discipline as including:

> the transfer of medical information (in audio, motion video, still images, graphics, text and other modalities) between distant locations with patients, physicians, other healthcare providers and medical institutions. It includes the use of telecommunication which links healthcare specialists with clinics, hospitals, primary physicians and patients in distant locations for diagnosis, treatment, consultations and continuing education.

Prehospital 'video triage' by a conferencing system allows the immediate assessment of an emergency situation. Many aspects of the physical examination can be performed remotely, such as applying a digital stethoscope to transmit the heart and breath sounds and other endoscopic devices to transmit physical information.

Digital output from echocardiography, ultrasonography, CT, and MRI equipment can be sent through a telemedicine link, allowing remote consultation between the emergency unit (remote or local) and a tertiary centre or radiology department. In addition, urgent laboratory reports can be transmitted together with the radiology report.

The most valuable contribution of PACS is the ability to integrate patients' past data, present images, and reports, and in enhancing storage and retrieval to make clinical care more efficient.

# CONCLUSION

The advent of newer techniques and the improvement of the currently available modalities will certainly have an impact in our future management of trauma patients. The array of new techniques may seem promising, allowing vast numbers of investigations to be performed readily, but it is prudent to obtain a balance between diagnostic choice and usefulness. Inherent risks or adverse effects from a particular new modality need to be constantly evaluated and fed back to manufacturers in order to secure new solutions and improvements.

# BIBLIOGRAPHY

Chait P. Future directions in interventional paediatric radiology. Pediatr Clin North Am 1997; 44(3):763–82.

Greene RE, Oestmann JW, eds. Computed Digital Radiography in Clinical Practice. New York: Thième Medical Publishers, 1992.

Krapichler C, Haubner M, Engelbrecht R, Englmeier KH. VR interaction techniques for medical imaging applications. Comput Methods Programs Biomed 1998; 56(1):65–74.

Krinsky G, Weinreb J. Gadolinum enhanced three dimensional MR angiography of the thoracoabdominal aorta. Semin Ultrasound CT MR 1996; 17(4):280–303.

Mallory D, McGee W, Shawker T, *et al*. Ultrasonic guidance improves the success rate of internal vein cannulation. Chest 1990; 98:157–60.

Melanson SW, Heller M. The emerging role of bedside ultrasonography in trauma care. Emerg Med Clin North Am 1998; 16(1):165–89.

Ohashi K, Brandser EA, el Khoury GY. Role of MR imaging in acute injuries to the appendicular skeleton. Radiol Clin North Am 1997; 35(3):591–613.

Reiser M, Faber SC. Recent and future advances in high speed imaging. Eur Radiol 1997; 7( Suppl. 5):166–73.

# *Useful measurements*

**Skull**
- Pituitary fossa — Height 6.5–11 mm; length 9–16 mm; breadth 9–19 mm
- Pineal gland shift (calcification) — ± 3 mm from the midline

**Neck/cervical spine**
- Pre-dental distance — Adult: 3 mm; Child: 5 mm
- C2 posterior displacement — <2 mm
- Physiological subluxation — C2/C3 (25%) and C3/C4 (15%) up to age 8 years
- Spinal canal sagittal diameter — 13 mm
- Prevertebral soft-tissue space — Adult: C1–C4 = 7 mm; C5–T1 = 22 mm
  Child: C1–C4 = 7 mm; C5–T1 = 14 mm
- Unstable cervical spine — Anterior displacement: > 3.5 mm with fracture >50% of the vertebra often indicates bilateral facet dislocation
  Compression fracture: >25% of the vertebral height
  Angulation: >11° between 2 vertebrae
  Facet joint space: >2 mm
- Compression fracture — Difference in anterior and posterior vertebral body height: >2 mm

**Thoracolumbar spine**
- Disc space — Disc space of L5/S1 = 2/3 of L4/L5
- Compression fracture — Difference in anterior and posterior vertebral body height: >2 mm (except T11–L1)
- Spinal burst fracture — Interpedicular or interspinous distance: >2 mm (between adjacent vertebra)

**Chest**
- ET tube — Tip: 5–7 cm from the carina; cuff = width of trachea
- Central line — Tip: junction of superior vena cava and right atrium
- Swan–Ganz catheter — Tip: main right or left proximal pulmonary artery
- Intra-aortic balloon pump — Tip: distal to left subclavian artery
- Superior mediastinum — <8 cm on upright film
- Diaphragm — Right higher than left hemidiaphragm up to 3 cm
- Hilum — Left hilum is higher than the right by 2 cm
- Nasogastric tube — Tip: within the stomach with side hole distal to gastrointestinal junction

**Upper Limb**
- Acromioclavicular joint — Distance: <8 mm; difference between sides: <3 mm
- Coracoid–clavicular distance — Distance: 11–13 mm; difference between sides: <5 mm
- Supinator fat strip — <1 cm
- Quadratus pronatus fat strip — <1 cm
- Radiocarpal joint — Radial angulation: 16°–28°; palmar angulation: 0°–22°; Radial length: 11–12 mm; radial shift: <1 mm
- Inferior radio-ulnar joint — <3 mm
- Scaphoid–lunate angle — 40°–70°
- Terry Thomas sign — >2 mm between scaphoid and lunate
- Metacarpal index — 5.4–7.9

*(Continued)*

**Pelvis**
- Pubic symphysis width            Normal: 7 mm; sacroiliac joint disruption > 2.5 cm

**Lower limb**
- Bohler's angle                   25°–40°
- Heel pad thickness               Males: <23 mm; females: <21.5 mm

# BIBLIOGRAPHY

Brunel W, Coleman DL, Schwartz DE, *et al.* Assessment of routine chest roentgenograms and the physical examination to confirm endotracheal tube position. Chest 1989; 96:1043.

Conrardy PA, Goodman LR, Lainge R, Singer MM. Alteration of endotracheal tube position: Flexion and extension of the neck. Crit Care Med 1976; 4:7.

Gilday DL. The value of chest radiography in the localisation of central venous pressure catheters. Can Med Assoc J. 1969; 101:363.

Hall WM, Rosenbaum HB. The radiology of cardiac pacemakers. Radiol Clin North Am 1971; 9:343.

Holger P, Han R. Measurements in Pediatric Radiology. Berlin: Springer Verlag, 1991.

Robert DR. Radiographic measurements. Philadelphia: JB Lippincott, 1989.

# Ossification centres

**Elbow**

| Ossification centre | Appears (approx. years) | Fuses (approx. years) |
|---|---|---|
| Capitellum | 2 | 17 |
| Radial head | 5 | 17 |
| Medial epicondyle | 5 | 17 |
| Trochlear | 10 | 18 |
| Olecranon | 11 | 18 |
| Lateral epicondyle | 12 | 18 |

**Wrist (carpal bones)**

| Ossification centre | Appears (approximate) |
|---|---|
| Capitate | birth |
| Hamate | 4 months |
| Triquetral | 3 years |
| Lunate | 4 years |
| Trapezium | 6 years |
| Trapezoid | 6 years |
| Scaphoid | 6 years |
| Pisiform | 10 years |

# Index